A CLINICAL MANUAL
OF PSYCHIATRY

A Clinical Manual Of Psychiatry

Edited by

Donald Oken, M.D.

Professor and Chairman
Department of Psychiatry, Upstate Medical Center
State University of New York, Syracuse, New York

and

Magnus Lakovics, M.D.

Assistant Professor and Director of Residency Training
Department of Psychiatry, Upstate Medical Center
State University of New York, Syracuse, New York

Elsevier / North-Holland
New York • Amsterdam • Oxford

Elsevier North Holland, Inc.
52 Vanderbilt Avenue, New York, New York 10017

Sole distributors outside the United States and Canada:
Elsevier Science Publishers B.V.
P.O. Box 211, 1000 AE Amsterdam, The Netherlands

Library of Congress Cataloging in Publication Data

Main entry under title:

A clinical manual of psychiatry.

    Bibliography: p.
    Includes index.
    1. Psychiatry—Handbooks, manuals, etc. I. Oken, Donald.
    II. Lakovics, Magnus. [DNLM: 1. Mental disorders.
    WM 100 0415c]
RC456.C57   616.89   81-12578
ISBN 0-444-00630-3   AACR2

Manufactured in the United States of America

To Our Wives
Linda and Eileen
Exemplars of Mental Health
and Essential to Ours

Contents

Preface

We have written this book to fill a void. Most textbooks of psychiatry have been written either for the beginner, who must acquire a broad orientation to the basic information and approach of the field, or the specialist, who needs to pursue particular issues in great depth. Very little is available for the physician or student who already has a general sense of the field of psychiatry but finds that the realities of clinical practice pose problems exceeding that knowledge, and who needs a source of reliable information that directly and usefully addresses those problems. This book is for them. It is not a textbook of psychiatry, but of *clinical* psychiatry. It addresses the major psychiatric problems seen in practice, and provides a sensible basis for the recognition, diagnosis, and treatment of those problems.

We believe it will have special usefulness for nonpsychiatrists, including those who work in "primary care" fields and in other clinical specialties. A large number of patients with psychiatric problems, likely a majority, are seen initially by these physicians; and many such patients appropriately receive continuing treatment from these same physicians. Residents in these fields, who see these same patients and should be developing their knowledge, will benefit also. Beginning psychiatric residents also may find it helpful. Their fund of practical knowledge at this stage usually is only a bit greater than trainees in other specialties, yet they are called upon as "instant experts" to deal with large numbers of the most acutely ill and difficult psychiatric patients. Finally, this book should prove helpful to those medical students who have already completed their basic work in psychiatry and are working in emergency rooms, medical clinics and wards, or in psychiatric units, beginning to confront the same problems that will later arise in residency and practice.

Most existing general psychiatric texts fall into two broad types. One is the complete textbook of psychiatry. This provides a thorough, detailed review of the basic sciences relevant to psychiatry; carefully considers the biological, psychological, and social factors involved in the various psychiatric disorders and problems; reviews their epidemiology, course, and outcome; and examines the nature of a variety of treatments as well as their applications to specific disorders. It meticulously explores theoretical and conceptual issues. Minor details and relatively obscure symptoms, disorders, and variants are considered carefully, despite their rarity, because of the light they may shed on theory or research. Such books are of great value. They provide beginning students with an appropriate breadth of view to develop a meaningful grasp of the new, puzzling conditions they are trying to understand. These are important also as source books to be consulted by the specialist or advanced student for additional detail, and to be mastered by the expert. They are to be carefully read, re-read, and digested.

For these very reasons, these books are not so helpful to a busy clinician. Often it is difficult to locate or identify specific information that has practical value relevant to a vexing clinical problem at hand or which recurs frequently, or to identify the key issues from a mass of intriguing but less relevant material.

Partly to deal with these shortcomings, another type of much shorter book has appeared, which covers psychiatry in a condensed fashion. In our experience, most of these have very limited usefulness. Many are literally "outlines" or close to that, dry as dust, which pander to the student who seeks a quick memory fix to pass an examination. Even were they readable, they represent "cookbooks" of facts which fail to do justice to the complex way in which patients present themselves. Nor can they provide the integrated picture a clinician needs to make a meaningful sense of clinical problems. Typically they merely boil down the longer texts into terse phrases and catchwords, while still trying to cover everything. Their lack of focus fails to meet the practical needs and priorities of clinical work. Those which avoid this trap do so by limiting themselves to certain types of clinical problems (for example, excluding major psychiatric disorders). But if a clinician already knew what he was dealing with, at least half his need for help would not exist. The problem is that typically he is uncertain about this and unclear about how to proceed to resolve that confusion.

Thus, this book takes a very different approach. While the overall range of coverage is broad, each chapter was written with an intensive, deliberate focus on these issues specifically relevant to clinical work.

The emphasis is selectively on material which is dependably established, not merely conjectural, and which is meaningful in clinical practice. To ensure that the priorities were based on the best available understanding of each disorder, we have assembled a group of authors who not only are recognized authorities about the conditions they describe, but clinicians working directly with patients who have these conditions. Each has provided a vivid, recognizable picture of the disorders and a sensible aproach to their diagnosis (and differential diagnosis) and their treatment, in practical terms. At the same time, each has taken pains to avoid an anti-intellectual dogmatism which would violate the complexity of clinical problems.

An effort has been made to maintain brevity consistent with the time pressures that physicians experience. But this has been achieved by eliminating less relevant material, not by providing outlines or recipes, or artificially preselecting coverage to a part of the clinical field. Care has been taken not to oversimplify the complexity of human beings and the psychiatric disorders they suffer, nor to portray these in unidimensional form. Whenever possible, clinical care is considered from an interactional (transactional) standpoint that emphasizes **the doctor–patient relationship as an unfolding two-person process.** Although we have limited ourselves to responding to the need of physicians for a brief source of useful information, we have tried to do so in a fashion that is consistent with the richness and intricacies of clinical work.

Although we were able to develop reasonable resolutions of the many technical problems posed in preparing this type of book, one has eluded us, except as we can deal with it here. We are fully aware that both doctors and patients are *shes* as well as *hes,* and acutely sensitive to the potential offensiveness of failing to refer to the former. At the same time, we are trapped by the realities of the English language: no alternative exists that is not impossibly awkward. With some reluctance, therefore, we have limited ourselves to the use of *he.*

We owe much to the great help of innumerable people in the labors that have led to this book—far too many to do more than mention more than the few most evident.

Clearly this book would not have seen the light of day without our contributors, who are listed in the following section. Not only are we grateful for the excellence of their chapters, but appreciative of their cooperation in adjusting their styles to maintain reasonable overall consistency throughout, despite intrinsic differences in the nature of the topics. We hope that they will forgive us for our badgering and carping to get details in place and to ensure that our publisher's deadlines were met. We thank them also for what they have taught us. In a very real sense, we were the first readers of this book and thus its first beneficiaries. We have learned much from them.

The forebearance, loyalty, and efficiency of our secretaries, Barbara Sullivan and Janet Miller, have been nothing short of remarkable. The translation of illegible handwriting into drafts and re-drafts, the checking and collating of manuscripts, and the obtaining and checking of references, were only the most visible part of their essential contributions. They managed to note our errors and to suggest corrections ever so tactfully, to guard our time jealously from outside intrusions, and, most difficult of all, to put up with our episodic temper tantrums and our irritability and idiosyncracies with incredible patience and cheerfulness. In addition to our own secretaries, everyone in our departmental secretarial staff was helpful in very many ways and deserves our thanks. But we are especially grateful to Barbara Svoboda, Mary Mc-Cargar, and Jacqueline McCoy, who carried out a number of burdensome extra tasks with extraordinary effectiveness.

We have been blessed also in our choice of publishers. The staff at Elsevier have been cooperative, tolerant, and helpful. They managed to strike a harmonious balance between being available when needed, yet never being intrusive. Their imput has been invaluable, yet they always made it clear that we had free rein in final decision making. Special acknowledgment is due to Louise Calabro Schreiber who worked closely with us to translate manuscripts into clear, readable chapters.

The number of teachers and colleagues who have indirectly contributed by educating us and helping us refine our thinking is literally beyond count, but we must pay special tributes to our students, especially our residents. Their curiosity, intellectual interest, good will, and forthrightness has heightened our awareness over the years of much that we did not know (but thought we did) and of paths that we might take to correct this.

Finally, our debt to our wives and families is immeasurable, beyond our capacity to express. In small compensation, this book is for them.

Donald Oken

Magnus Lakovics

Contributors

Anthony E. Blumetti, Ph.D.
Assistant Professor, Division of Clinical Psychology, Department of Psychiatry, and Consultant, Pain Treatment Service, State University Hospital, State University of New York Upstate Medical Center, Syracuse, New York.

Robert Cancro, M.D., Med. D. Sc.
Professor and Chairman, Department of Psychiatry, New York University Medical Center, New York, New York.

Gene D. Cohen, M.D.
Chief, Center for Studies of the Mental Health of the Aging, National Institute of Mental Health, Rockville, Maryland.

Sidney Cohen, M.D.
Clinical Professor of Psychiatry, Neuropsychiatric Institute, UCLA Center for the Health Sciences, Los Angeles, California, and Editor, *The Drug Abuse and Alcoholism Newsletter.*

Leon Eisenberg, M.D.
Maude and Lillien Presley Professor of Social Medicine and Professor of Psychiatry, and Chairman, Department of Social Medicine and Health Policy, Harvard Medical School, and Senior Associate in Psychiatry, Children's Hospital Medical Center, Boston, Massachusetts.

Anthony Kales, M.D.
Professor and Chairman, Department of Psychiatry, and Director, Sleep Research and Treatment Center, Pennsylvania State University, Hershey, Pennsylvania.

Joyce D. Kales, M.D.
Associate Professor, Department of Psychiatry, and Associate Director, Sleep Research
and Treatment Center, Pennsylvania State University, Hershey, Pennsylvania.

Eugene A. Kaplan, M.D.
Associate Professor, and Director, Behavioral Science Program, Department of
Psychiatry, State University of New York Upstate Medical Center, Syracuse, New
York.

Gerald L. Klerman, M.D.
Professor of Psychiatry, Harvard Medical School, and Director, Stanley Cobb
Psychiatric Research Laboratories, Massachusetts General Hospital, Boston,
Massachusetts.

Magnus Lakovics, M.D.
Assistant Professor, and Director of Residency Training, Department of Psychiatry,
State University of New York Upstate Medical Center, Syracuse, New York.

John C. Nemiah, M.D.
Professor of Psychiatry, Harvard Medical School, and Psychiatrist-in-Chief, Beth Israel
Hospital, Boston, Massachusetts.

Donald Oken, M.D.
Professor and Chairman, Department of Psychiatry, State University of New York
Upstate Medical Center, Syracuse, New York.

Donald M. Pirodsky, M.D.
Assistant Professor, Department of Psychiatry, State University of New York Upstate
Medical Center, and Director, Consultation-Liaison Service, and Staff Psychiatrist,
Syracuse VA Medical Center, Syracuse, New York.

Franklin G. Reed, M.D.
Clinical Assistant Professor, Department of Psychiatry, State University of New York
Upstate Medical Center, Syracuse, New York.

David A. Waller, M.D.
Associate Professor of Psychiatry and Pediatrics, and Director, Pediatric–Psychiatry
Liaison Service, Southwestern Medical School, University of Texas Health Science
Center at Dallas, Dallas, Texas.

A Note on DSM III

In 1980, the American Psychiatric Association issued the new, 3rd edition of the *Diagnostic and Statistical Manual of Mental Disorders (DSM III)*. This document represents the official version of the diagnostic system applicable to all mental disorders and related conditions (for psychiatry in the United States). It embodies a major departure from the prior two official diagnostic systems. The changes include the utilization of a multiaxial system of diagnoses and specific descriptive diagnostic criteria for each diagnosis, as well as a new classification system which includes modifications and regroupings of the previous diagnostic categories.

The **multiaxial approach** provides a comprehensive, clinically relevant diagnostic picture by going beyond the conventional specification of the primary disorder alone to include other important factors. *Axis I* is used for the standard clinical diagnosis. The presence of any underlying personality disorder or developmental disorder is indicated on *Axis II*. *Axis III* specifies any current physical disorder or condition which may be relevant to the understanding or management of the patient. In addition, the severity of the relevant psychosocial stressors *(Axis IV)* and the highest prexisting level of adaptive functioning *(Axis V)* may be specified optionally. Thus complete multiaxial diagnosis places a psychiatric illness within a broader context that is more meaningful in understanding the situation of the patient as a whole.

Explicit **diagnostic criteria** are listed for each disorder. These include features that are so characteristic as to be essential for a diagnosis, and those typical of the disorder, especially in aggregate. In addition, findings or other diagnoses which exclude the given diagnosis are specified. The criteria are descriptive, verifiable, overt behavioral phenomena: primarily signs and symptoms plus age and durational factors. Underlying psychological processes are excluded as criteria, by intent.

Correspondingly, the organization of the **classification system** is based on overt behavior, purposefully eschewing psychodynamic or other psychological principles. The stated intent is that the system be "atheoretical," while compatible with all theoretical systems. It has been pointed out, however, that the descriptive behavioral approach is, to some extent, a theoretical position per se, which has influenced both the classification scheme and the naming of disorders in ways that are not entirely congenial to a psychodynamic orientation. For the most part, these objections do not pose a serious problem to the concomitant use of both approaches.

With regard to the neuroses, however, this problem has been more troublesome, and the greatest source of controversy about the "correctness" of DSM III. The psychodynamic approach emphasizes the underlying unity of these disorders: thus their inclusion within the single rubric of neuroses. But DSM III fragments this grouping, assigning various neuroses to different parts of the classification schema, sometimes grouped disorders which are psychodynamically different, although behaviorally similar. For example conversion disorder (hysterical neuroses, conversion type) is grouped with other disorders having primarily somatic symptoms, including hypochondriasis; and is in a category separate from other varieties of hysterical neurosis, e.g., psychogenic fugue and psychogenic amnesia.

Use of DSM III in This Book

The descriptions of the clinical disorders and of their relationship with other conditions (their place in the classification scheme) is **compatible with DSM III throughout this book.** The reader should have no difficulty applying the information here to making a DSM III diagnosis for any patient.

The only places where this is apparently not so is Chapter 8, on the neuroses. This is organized in terms of DSM II for reasons explained in that chapter. But even there, the descriptions of the disorders are consistent with DSM III, and the relationship of the earlier and new classification systems is made explicit. Elsewhere, there is occasional use of terms belonging to a variety of older classifications because these have explanatory value, but within the context of DSM III categories.

Nevertheless, the material in this book is far from being the same as that included in DSM III. The emphasis of DSM III is on classification and the delineation of criterion lists for every diagnostic category. The discussions in this book represent integrated descriptions of the way the various major conditions unfold and display themselves to the clinicians who must recognize and make sense of them. This is no "book of lists." Rather than analyze the threads making up the rich tapestry of clinical psychiatry, the emphasis is on the pictures portrayed. Practical issues in eliciting and organizing clinical data also are emphasized. And, of course, so is treatment.

For the convenience of the reader, a summary of the DSM III classification that lists all the Axis I and II diagnostic categories is provided in the Appendix.

A CLINICAL MANUAL
OF PSYCHIATRY

PART I

THE DIAGNOSTIC PROCESS

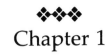

Chapter 1

The Doctor–Patient Relationship:
The Diagnostic Interview

Donald Oken

We start this book with a consideration of the doctor–patient relationship because we must. That is the beginning. It is the foundation on which all of clinical psychiatry rests, as does all of clinical medicine.

The centrality of this relationship for medicine rests on an understanding that patients—all human beings—are "bio-psycho-social" entities. This is a somewhat cumbersome way of indicating that mind (psyche) and body (soma) represent an integrated whole in constant interaction with the environment, social as well as biological; and that **all** must be considered in a unified fashion, if any is to be understood effectively. That seems a cliche, easily espoused but often ignored. Doctors may act as if they were treating diseases. But for the physician, **there are no diseases which occur "in" people, there are only dis-eased (sick) people** (patients). The doctor, equally a person, relates to a patient to change the latter's state to one of well-being, or at least in that direction.

Modern biomedical science has made advances that are little less than incredible. However, its insights have tended to be perverted in their application, as if sick people were inanimate particles in a test tube. Complaints about depersonalized medicine are increasingly heard. As an antidote, many have emphasized a need for greater humanism: more kindness and caring for the patient. Unfortunately, this misses the point, being based on the same error as the problem it seeks to alleviate. This "holistic" or "humanistic" view approaches the problem as if the issue were one merely of ethics, rather than one of science as well. It implies that we should be humane to people **while** we treat their diseases. The dichotomy is perpetuated.

There can be no argument that it is ethically good for physicians to behave in a thoroughly humane manner. But beyond this, **it is a scientific fact that treating a sick person as such, and not "a disease," is therapeutically more effective.** Patients respond better. They become well faster. One need not substitute humanism for science.

It is in the unfolding nature of the two-person, doctor–patient relationship that treatment occurs: a therapeutic alliance that encompasses biological, psychological, and social factors.

Neither doctor nor patient come to their relationship as newborn babes. Each has a pattern of expectancies laid down in their respective personal and sociocultural backgrounds. Much of this background is shared, although it is always colored by individual differences in experience and personality.

The patient comes with a wish for help and the anticipation he will get it. The patient is fearful and concerned both about his symptoms and what they may mean: what dread disease may be causing them (concerns which tend to run especially high in the psychiatric patient). The patient hopes and expects that the doctor will make him feel better— and get better. These feelings center on the physician's technical expertise, of course. But they have other potent determinants. Their roots lie in the predominantly positive, lifelong experience with caregivers, originally the parents. Just as a parent's hugs and tender reassurances comfort a hurt child, patients with a coronary have reported feeling less pain and concern immediately following a telephone conversation with the doctor, secure in the knowledge that his help is on the way. The decrease in pain and anxiety reduces the strain on the heart: an actual therapeutic result.

Most patients come primed largely with good feelings and hope. But no one has escaped bad experiences entirely nor lacks the knowledge that even good treatment often hurts. Hence, a readiness for fearful, hurt, and angry feelings coexist.

The doctor is also invested with the mantle of the magician–priest (who is the doctor in primitive societies). There is much about medical treatment and its settings that are strange, complex, and wondrous, to the point of awe. This too is a double-edged sword: on one hand, promoting expectation of magical cure; on the other, dread and the potential for rage at the magician caught tricking us, revealing himself a charlatan.

The doctor–patient relationship is so unique and so important that it has special status, codified in law and embodied in social convention. **The doctor's role** is defined to include the power to have a patient reveal both his nude body and most secret thoughts, and to inflict pain and even injury (surgery) on the patient. But with this license come obligations: to respect the patient's person and his revelations, and to use these only in his work for the patient; to hurt safely and only in the service of treatment; and to be competent. It is this combination of attributes that we refer to as the doctor's professional behavior.

In return, the sick person assumes the **patient role.** He is obliged to reveal himself, and put himself in the hands of the doctor, behaviors which are charged with ambivalence. With this, he gains permission to reveal his guilty secrets with safety and absolution, to receive treatment, and to be dependent and have the privileged exemptions of the sick from certain social responsibilities. (It is okay to stay home and take it easy once the doctor says you are "sick.")

It is the doctor's behavior that determines how successfully this relationship, with its "role-complementarity," will function. Its success rests on his capacity to demonstrate that he does, in fact, respect the patient and his confidences, is gentle and concerned, and acts with competence. To accomplish this in the face of the fears and suspicions always latent in the patient (especially the psychiatric patient) requires that the doctor deal effectively with the obstructions derived from the patient's experience and personality. He must tolerate, work around, or, where necessary, modify these negative influences. This depends upon his capacity to empathize with or transcend those aspects of the patient's background and reactions to the doctor that arise as interferences.

The Psychiatric Patient

In developing the relationship with the psychiatric patient, the doctor faces special challenges. These patients tend to have high levels of anxiety, guilt, shame, and other dysphoric feelings which become heightened by assuming the patient role. Many of them have had unsatisfactory experiences with prior caregivers, including those physicians who were put off by their behavioral symptoms. In some instances, relationships with others have never been good, going back to those with their parents. Thus, their capacity to allow or sustain trust is likely to be fragile. Whether cause or effect of their disturbed state, regression is a common feature, resulting in immature behavior, with unreasonable demands on the doctor and an overreaction to their inevitable frustration.

To the extent that these nonspecific problems exist, the doctor's most helpful response is an extra measure of patience and demonstration of his gentleness and dependability. **Taking the patient's concerns seriously, as legitimate and distressing symptoms,** strengthens trust. Calmness works to allay anxiety (and vice versa). Tacit or overt reassurances about confidentiality are especially important, not only because of exaggerated guilt and shame, but also because very intimate details of personal life may be issues in the illness. Regressive behavior during the examination is usually best met with an attitude of firm kindness ("tough, but oh so gentle"). This is not unlike the appropriate response of a good parent to an upset child; although pains must be taken to convey respect and to avoid the patronizing message that the doctor thinks of the patient as a child. And, of course, listening for and hearing what it is that concerns the patient is crucial, as with every patient.

This is often easier than it may seem. Psychiatric patients are greatly upset by a layman's reactions to their symptoms as bizarre, unacceptable, repugnant, or frightening. But the doctor who recognizes that these are symptoms, not moral defects, usually finds that the patient soon begins to relate satisfactorily and provide a useful history; indeed, the symptoms may abate in the process.

Patients in a rage are permitted to ventilate freely (even at the doctor) and offered statements of empathic understanding of their feelings, but never allowed to behave destructively. (If behavioral control is deficient, additional help is summoned at once. Often its mere presence will suffice.) The persecutory or grandiose ideas of a paranoid patient are accepted. Their reality is never directly challenged. But sympathetic questions may be raised about the experiences giving rise to these. One may laugh sparingly with a manic patient, but never at him. Misperceptions and confusions about the immediate situation, once fully identified, are best corrected in simple, direct fashion, as if they are a source of interference or continuing anxiety. These and other details of management of particular disorders are considered in greater depth in the chapters on each.

The Diagnostic Interview

The initial doctor–patient contact serves two purposes concomitantly. It establishes the doctor–patient relationship, and uses this as a vehicle to obtain "the history"—information needed to determine diagnosis and treatment.

Too often, the former process is regarded as superfluous, or even an interference to the data-gathering task. In fact, the way the doctor conducts this interview determines not merely the nature of the subsequent relationship, but the quality of the historical information. The degree to which the relationship is perceived progressively as a secure, professional one determines what and how much the patient will choose to reveal. Humane though it may be, the skillful interview represents the application of behavioral science to quality medical care. The capacity to interview well is a matter of technical expertise, honed by practice. It depends on a knowledge of the features of interpersonal communication, as well as insight, derived from psychology and the social sciences, into the meaning of the information provided by the patient.

Recognition of this has led to renaming the process of history taking as the medical, or diagnostic, **interview.** This term reflects more accurately the fact that two people are involved in an interaction,[1] each of whom is viewing the other. Both are evolving viewpoints about the other and their relationship. What each person communicates at any moment reflects the status of these perceptions. The term interview also avoids the implication that the activity is one-sided (the doctor "taking" something—the history—from the patient), with the added connotation that the process is adversarial. Both parties are constantly shaping their relationship in terms of what has transpired, as well as the expectancies each has brought to the situation. For the reasons already given, usually this is cooperative, though how effectively so depends upon the doctor's interviewing skills.

The doctor should make the initial interview as complete as possible. This may not be necessary simply to "make the diagnosis." **The objective is to understand the patient.** This broader knowledge will be of continuing value as the treatment continues, as well as establishing the point that it is the sick person in whom the doctor is interested, not simply his disease.

This initial session is optimum for another reason. A patient comes to a doctor because he hurts in some way. His level of pain and concern is likely highest at this point in time. Consequently, so is the pressure of his motivation to be self-revealing. As he begins later to feel better, he is increasingly likely to censor what seems to him unnecessary or trivial. He may "forget" to mention that his depression was preceded by a job promotion, a fight with his wife, or the death of a beloved aunt. Yet these bits of information are crucial to diagnosis and understanding the person. The doctor who conducts a thorough interview initially capitalizes on the occasion when the patient's motivation to reveal personal information is at its peak.

The formal tradition of beginning the history with the "chief complaint" followed by the "present illness" relates to this same point. Obviously, these usually provide key diagnostic clues. But they also are what the patient wants most to talk about: how he hurts. Their priority is felt mutually, if for different reasons.

In emergencies, perhaps little more than these data can be obtained. Patients in panic, paralyzed by depressive retardation, or struggling with psychotic disorganization—just as those with crushing substernal pain and dyspnea—are in no condition to provide more. Nor can their treatment wait upon it. Such situations parallel that of the pediatrician with young children, and approach that of the veterinarian. The doctor

---

[1]Technically, this is a transaction rather than an interaction; but the commonsense term is adequate.

is forced to convey his concern and regard for the patient within the limitations of his limited inquiry and conduct of the examination. Other information is obtained from family and friends. But the physician who does not return for a thorough interview when his patient's condition permits, limits his capacities to that of the veterinarian. And he communicates to the patient that his interest, kindly though it may be, is akin to that he might show to a dumb animal.

What the doctor needs to know beyond this, in terms of the various categories of history (past, family and personal history, and the like) is generally well covered in medical education, and widely appreciated. Reminders of those aspects specifically pertinent to each of the major psychiatric disorders, as well as to the conduct of the mental status examination, are covered in subsequent chapters.

It might be noted, however, that very little of the mental status "examination" ever needs to be performed as a separate activity. This is yet another fringe benefit for the physician who interviews well and listens carefully. A good diagnostic interview intrinsically provides most of what needs to be known about the patient's mental status. All that remains is to fill in a few residual areas of ambiguity or missing data, and to confirm leads in more systematic depth.

How the interview is conducted is far less well known. Good technique is rarely taught adequately; and its value is insufficiently appreciated. Yet, once the investment in learning to do this is made, it pays continuing dividends.

The key point is that **only the patient knows and can relate his "history."** Obviously, he is the one who possesses the facts. Less obviously, he is the only one who can make the connections that clarify sequences, link symptoms to life events, or reveal the meanings of such events. Most of this is revealed in what is said. The remainder comes from the order in which it is told, the descriptive terms used, the concomitant gestures and facial expressions, and what has obviously been left unsaid. For this reason, **the major task of the interviewing physician is to facilitate the patient's reporting of events in the patient's own words.** Secondarily, the doctor helps the patient reveal what is pertinent by defining relevant areas or topics. But this too is largely a product of leads provided by the patient.

The main job is to keep the patient talking spontaneously, indicating, when necessary, those areas which require amplification and more precise detail. Much of this is done via the seeming simplicity of encouraging nods and vocal reinforcements ("uh huh. . . ?") or repetitions of phrases and words originally used by the patient. This is supplemented by broad, open-ended questions. ("Tell me more about those 'strange thoughts' "; "What was your 'funny mood' like?") Use of the patient's own words minimizes the subtle introduction of the doctor's premature assumptions, which can falsely color the story. When the time is appropriate, the doctor introduces new areas of enquiry. Again, this is done in as **open-ended** a way as possible, permitting the patient to convey what is pertinent. ("Have you ever had fears like this before?"; "Now I'd like to know something about your family.") Only at the end of the coverage of a topical area are specific questions raised. These are, of course, necessary to fill in specific details. But, wherever possible, these are asked in such a way as to make other than a yes/no answer possible, giving the patient the opportunity to provide an unforeseen detail.

Great care is taken to avoid expressions of the doctor's personal opinions, values, or judgments. At best these are irrelevant. More than likely, they will define for the patient what he dare not reveal. Worse, they taint the whole relationship with the fear that broader censorship is necessary. The doctor has enough problems with the censorship motivated by the patient's intrinsic guilt, fear, and embarrassment to add yet other inhibitions. Nor can he afford to undermine the precious sense of alliance which it is his prime task to cultivate.

This neutrality has other advantages. It permits us to get an undistorted picture of how the patient relates to us: its style as well as its quality. This becomes a clue to how he relates to similar others in his life. (A patient who constantly corrects the most minor, irrelevant details, to the point of distraction, is likely to be perceived as no less annoying by his acquaintances.) It helps establish the diagnosis (in the example just given, a possible compulsive personality disorder). And it portends the way the patient will respond to particular treatment modes. (An overmeticulous person is likely to respond better to a scheduled regimen of medication than one offered on a p.r.n. basis.)

This interview technique is at once simpler and more difficult than it seems. The doctor does as little as possible—overtly. But unobtrusively he is constantly at work, listening actively while stimulating the patient to talk productively. This subtle, active work also protects the interview from wandering afield or becoming bogged down in repetitions or minutiae. Fears that use of his method will consume too much time represent a misunderstanding that the doctor is just passively listening. Once the full basic picture has been painted in the patient's own manner and words, the doctor moves expeditiously to deflect tangential, garrulous talk by maneuvers which get the patient back on the track. ("Let's see, you were telling me about 'being followed by communists' "; "Please tell me now about your job"; "You said that you live with your parents?")

It is true that the process takes longer than the type of interview one conducts in an emergency, which is designed at getting just the immediately essential "facts." But this is because one gets many more pertinent facts. This approach recognizes that the facts needed go be-

yond a bare-bones symptomatic report, to gain an understanding of the
ill person. As a consequence, diagnosis becomes both more accurate and
more meaningful.

Paradoxically, the well-conducted complete interview even pays dividends in time. When the doctor who has hurriedly taken an inadequate
history realizes he needs additional information, he finds it takes much
more time to get it than originally; and he will almost surely get it less
well and less easily. An initial interview is the most efficient and eco-
nomical. The truncated interview conducted in emergencies merely
seems more efficient. A little reflection reveals that it often provides false
leads, requires supplementation by family or others, and makes extra
laboratory work necessary. These make the total process longer. Moreover, all this reveals barely enough data to manage the immediate situation, not enough for treating the patient.

Time spent initially also expedites treatment. The positive relationship
established has a potent therapeutic effect in itself. Moreover, it promotes the cooperation and compliance that come with the patient's commitment to the therapeutic alliance. Powerful treatment effects have
been instituted from the first possible moment.

By far the most common complaint about doctors today is that we fail
to communicate. We fail to listen enough. We cut off anything beyond
the supposed facts or regard it as irrelevancy to which we need not
attend. Patients are not allowed to explain, nor unburden themselves
of the concerns that actually have brought them. We leave them with
unspoken or unanswered questions. We hurry past these or close discussion with answers to their surface meanings, failing to respond in
an open-ended way that probes for what lies beneath, which they really
want to know.

Those who misperceive this complaint as "consumerism" miss the
point. It cannot be resolved by a slicker bedside manner, better public
relations, or even more kindness. It is a concern that touches on our
skill in interviewing and developing the doctor–patient relationship,
which is based on the science of human behavior. This skill is the most
fundamental and most central clinical tool in medicine.

Additional Readings

Bowden CL, Burstein AG: Psychosocial Basis of Medical Practice. Baltimore,
    Williams & Wilkins, 1974, Part 1, pp 3–81

MacKinnon RA, Michels R: The Psychiatric Interview in Clinical Practice. Phil-
    adelphia, WB Saunders, 1971, Chapter 1, pp 3–64

Morgan WL, Engel GL: The Clinical Approach to the Patient. Philadelphia, WB
    Saunders, 1969, Chapters 1–3, pp 1–79

Stevenson I: The Psychiatric Interview, in American Handbook of Psychiatry,
    2nd ed., vol. 1. Edited by Arieti S. New York, Basic Books, 1974, Chapter 53,
    pp 1138–1156

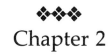

Chapter 2

The Mental Status Examination

Magnus Lakovics

The *mental status examination* is done by interview and observation; by means of it, data are obtained and organized in a special form to give specific information about all major aspects of mental functioning. It is often asked whether that examination is a separate process, or if it represents only information obtained from the regular history and physical examination. Part of the confusion arises because the mental status examination is always written and presented separately from the remainder of the workup. The answer depends on how much information about the patient's mental status is obtained during the usual interview. Three possibilities exist: all, some, or little information is obtained for a complete mental status examination during that routine interview. If less than complete information is obtained, then a more or less involved formal separate mental status examination will have to be done at the end of the routine interview. The extent of this separate examination depends both on the patient's problem and the experience of the interviewer. For example, a depressed patient may express suicidal thoughts during the course of history taking. But if he fails to do so, he must later be asked specifically about suicide. An experienced physician hearing a subtle reference to "seeing things" during a routine interview, will pursue this to clarify whether the patient is hallucinating. But a less-experienced one may miss this cue in his routine interview; he must therefore always ask about "seeing things" in a later separate review of the patient's mental status, or he may miss the diagnosis entirely. For the inexperienced physician, it is almost always best to do a separate formal mental status examination in evaluating any patient in whom a possible psychiatric disorder may exist.

Table 1

OBSERVATION
  Appearance
    Dress
    Grooming
    Facial expression
    Bodily movements, motor behavior
    Interpersonal relating

LISTENING, QUESTIONING, AND TESTING
  Speech
    Content
    Rate, volume, flow
    Emotional tone, expressiveness, appropriateness
  Thought
    Process
      Disturbances in structure of associations—word salad, tangentiality,
        circumstantiality, neologism, perseveration, condensation, incoherence or
        looseness, irrelevant answers
      Disturbances in speed of association—flight of ideas, clang associations, blocking
    Content
      Homicidal or suicidal ideation
      Delusional thinking, other preoccupations
    Perceptual Disturbances
      Hallucinations
      Illusions
    Cognitive Function
      Level of consciousness
      Orientation to time, place, person
      Calculating ability
      Memory: immediate retention, recent and remote recall
      Fund of knowledge, vocabulary
      Abstracting ability
      Judgment and insight

SELF- AND OTHER-AWARENESS
  Patient's effect upon the examiner
  Patient's response to the examiner

Obtaining the necessary data for a complete mental status examination can be separated into three tasks: (1) observation, (2) listening, questioning and testing and (3) exploring self- and other-awareness. The data to be obtained through each of these three tasks are summarized in Table 1.

Observation

Observation begins when the patient is first seen. Much can be gleaned from **appearance.** Dress tells us a good deal. Is it appropriate to the situation, reasonably neat, harmonious, and in keeping with the patient's socioeconomic status? For example, an extremely bright, able, well-dressed man was seen in the emergency room. The examiner could not ascertain the patient's difficulty but noticed that the patient was wearing sneakers with his pinstriped, three-piece, vested suit. Although initially an acute anxiety disorder was suspected, further examination revealed a well-hidden paranoid psychosis. Disparate dress can be one of the first indicators of psychological decompensation.

Grooming is important. An unkempt business executive may be experiencing acute depression, whereas a construction worker may look unkempt because he simply did not stop at home to change.

Facial expressions convey much about the patient's mood and emotionality. A furrowed brow can be a sign of depression. An expressionless face may indicate blunted or flattened affect. Excessive smiling and laughing may be the beginning of a manic episode. Smiling when talking about a major life tragedy indicates inappropriate affect. Facial grimacing suggests movement disorder or schizophrenia.

Bodily movements and other motor behavior similarly can give us information about the patient's mood, neurological functioning, social habits, and level of anxiety. Rapid pacing may represent anxiety or panic. A gesturing patient may be "warding off the evil eye" or trying to locate the source of a draft in the room. A patient who stands rigid and immobile without talking may be catatonic. Slowed movements suggest psychomotor retardation (depression).

Observation of **interpersonal relating** gives much information about personality as well as psychological functioning. A patient who avoids eye contact throughout the interview, and gives a vague, poorly detailed history that omits mention of any significant people in his life, may be looking for help from schizoid avoidance. On the other hand, an alluring and seductive woman may appear to be quite well adjusted; but within this facade she may be very troubled and conflicted because of her inability to control her impulsiveness. Finally, a schizophrenic patient who ignores social custom in relation to bodily distance may stand disturbingly close to the examiner, thus illustrating the fearful chaos inside.

Listening, Questioning and Testing

The **content, rate, volume, flow, and emotional tone of speech** are indicators of many aspects of current functioning. Illogical content may be an indication of schizophrenic loosening of associations, or "word salad." Disordered pronunciation may represent dysarthria. Words which are omitted or misused to describe objects may be indicative of aphasia. Speech which is so rapid as to be difficult to comprehend may be a result of manic flight of ideas. Someone who speaks louder than is necessary may be deaf or manic. Difficulty in finding the right word may be schizophrenic blocking or the speech of the foreign-born. Talking without inflection may be indicative of the flatness of the schizophrenic's life.

With the psychoses, personality and depressive disorders, it is essential to ask directly whether the patient has ever thought of hurting himself or others.

Delusional thinking is defined as a fixed false belief not amenable to reason. Usually this is revealed during the history, but will not be evident unless the examiner thoroughly pursues leads given by the patient. For example:

PATIENT: They always make me think.

EXAMINER: Who does?

PATIENT: The people in the building up there.

EXAMINER: Which building?

PATIENT: You know, the one where they have all those TV sets and programs.

EXAMINER: How do they do this?

PATIENT: They make me think thoughts through those TV sets.

Disturbance in the structure and speed of associations may not appear if the examiner is too directive in his interview. A patient with mild disturbance in association may be able to answer questions which require brief, concrete answers, and never demonstrate the disturbance. Thus, questions like, "Are you married?"; "Where do you live?"; "How many children do you have?"; "When did your problems begin?"; and "How long have you been having these problems?" will generally not elicit disturbances in the structure of association. In contrast, questions like, "What is your wife like?"; "Can you describe your children to me?"; "Please tell me what it was like for you when your problems began," etc., stimulate responses involving sentences which tax thought organization and association. In general, it is best to ask the unstructured questions first to illustrate the disturbance in the structure and speed of associations, and then to ask more structured questions in order to obtain necessary additional data.

Disturbances in **perception,** like those in association, often are elicited in the course of the history taking. But, if visual or auditory hallucinations, or illusory phenomena are not described, it is best to ask the patient directly if he is seeing visions, has disturbances in seeing things, or hears voices. On occasion, an entire history and mental status examination may be done without much evidence of psychotic thought process (particularly in well-defended paranoid schizophrenic patients) unless these questions are asked **specifically.**

Disturbances in **cognitive function** may show up when the patient (or his family) comments that he tends to forget things. It may even be obvious from the patient's verbalizations; for example, an elderly patient, retired for many years, may say, "I'm sorry, Doctor, but I have to go to work now." Even when the diagnosis of an organic mental disorder is obvious, its severity and pervasiveness must be defined. And in more subtle cases, such as early mild gradual dementia, the signs may not be apparent without formal testing. Formal testing of cognitive function can be done at the end of history taking with a statement like, "I'm going to ask you some questions. Some may be more difficult than others, and some may seem foolish. Just answer them as best as you can." The examiner can then proceed to ask the patient his full name, where he is, and the date. **Calculating ability** can be tested by requesting the patient to do simple addition and subtraction or to count backwards from a hundred by 7's: "7 from 100 is 93 and 7 from 93 is . . . ?" **Immediate retention** can be tested by requesting the patient to repeat numbers given by the examiner forward and backward. Patients with organic mental disorders generally can repeat numbers forward much better than backward. Most unimpaired patients should be able to repeat five to six digits forward, and four to five backward.

Asking a patient to remember and repeat three objects after two minutes, such as red, table, 63 Broadway, can also be useful. However, in drawing conclusions from the results of repetition of numbers and objects, it is necessary to keep in mind that these activities correlate with intelligence and may not be a primary function of memory. **Recent recall** can be determined by questions such as, "How did you get to the hospital?"; "What did you have for lunch today?" etc. To be certain of the answers, it may be necessary to check with an accompanying family member or other person. Accurateness of remote recall is usually apparent from the history, and may, if necessary, be correlated with data obtained from accompanying persons. The most useful tests in differentiating organic from functional psychiatric illness are recall of remote personal events or recent general events (Manschreck and Keller, 1979). **Fund of knowledge** as well as recall for recent general events can usually be ascertained by broadening questioning to include such things as current or well-known historical events. Questions can also be asked directly which test this knowledge, such as, "Can you tell me the last five presidents?"; and "Who is the governor of your state?" **Abstracting ability** can be tested through the use of proverbs. The patients should be able to respond to a proverb such as, "Don't cry over spilled milk" with a statement like, "Everbody makes mistakes"; "You shouldn't let it get you down"; or "What's done is done." If a patient personalizes proverbs as in "My cat spills milk," or concretizes, as in "Spilled milk is messy," this may be an indicator of poor abstracting ability due to a schizophrenic thought disorder or brain syndrome.

Finally, **judgment and insight** are best ascertained from the interview and responses to questions about the patient's difficulties, daily living and/or behavior. Questions like, "What would you do if you found an addressed, stamped envelope in the street?"; "What would you do if you were in a crowded movie theater and smelled smoke?" have also been used in forming an overall impression about judgment although their usefulness has recently been challenged (Manschreck and Keller, 1979). **Insight,** in the limited sense of a mental status examination, means that a patient is aware of having problems and recognizes the impact of the difficulties on his functioning.

Self- and Other-Awareness

The mental status examination, like the physical examination, is a dyadic process in which both participants have an effect on one another. We are examining not only the patient but also the reactions elicited by the patient, which also provide information about his mental status. One unique aspect of bio-psycho-social processes in humans is that what we observe often changes because of the impact we have through our movement, feelings, observation, verbal, and nonverbal communication with the patient. For example, a patient's anxiety may escalate if we feel anxious about examining him. Similarly, paranoia may increase if we are secretive. A hysterical patient may act more seductively if our attraction is conveyed. Our impact on the patient and our reactions to him are important data, provided we see them as such, and use them to interpret and understand him, rather than merely reacting, thereby distorting our powers of observation.

Drawing Conclusions

Once the examiner has accomplished the tasks of observation, listening, questioning, testing, and exploring awareness, and has recorded data obtained in these tasks, the mental status examination can then be considered complete. Table 2 summarizes and defines the common signs and symptoms of psychiatric disorders.

As elsewhere in medicine, accurate diagnosis cannot be made on the examination alone, but must include historical data as well. Furthermore, the presence of any given sign or symptom can be very misleading out of context. This is more true for mental than physical findings, since disturbance of one function may distort another. For example, in cases of acute psychosis, because of much agitation and fear our questions related to orientation may not be heard and answered. Yet orientation may be intact and may be revealed only after the patient is calmed. Or findings of inappropriate affect, loosening of associations, hallucina-

Table 2. Common Signs and Symptoms of Psychiatric Disorders

THOUGHT	
Looseness of association and incoherence	Sentence not logical—one phrase in a sentence not logically following another, incomprehensibility
Circumstantiality and tangentiality	Inability to speak to the point, wandering thought content, sentences still comprehensible
Neologism	Creating new words
Echolalia	Repeating the words of another person
Perseveration	Repetitively using a word or phrase in response to different questions
Flight of ideas	Rapid flow of ideas, one immediately following another
Blocking	Stopping in mid-sentence or between sentences and not being able to continue
Clang association	Expression of thoughts stimulated by words sounding similar but not meaning the same thing
Delusion	Fixed, false belief
Obsession	Persistence of a thought or feeling not able to be eliminated by conscious will

AFFECT	
Inappropriate	Emotions not consonant with the content of speech and thought (e.g., smiling when talking about death of a close friend)
Flat or blunted	Absence or markedly diminished display of any feelings generally
Predominant or extreme	Anxiety, depression, elation, etc.
Lability	Rapidly fluctuating emotions

LEVEL OF ACTIVITY	
Hyperactivity	Excessive, sometimes aggressive activity
Compulsivity	Repeating an act because of an uncontrollable urge
Hypoactivity	Slowing of activity, e.g., psychomotor retardation, catatonia
Echopraxia	Repeating the movements of another person

(*continued*)

Table 2 *(continued)*

SENSORIUM	
Distractibility	Inability to concentrate or screen out background stimuli
Disorientation	Loss of time, place, or person sense
Level of consciousness	Clouding of consciousness, inability to maintain attention
Cognitive dysfunction	Loss of memory and intellectual abilities, (e.g., judgment, calculation, abstract thought)
PERCEPTION	
Hallucination (auditory, visual, tactile, etc.)	Perception not based on a realistic external stimulus
Illusion	Distorted perception of a real external stimulus

tions, and disorientation in an adolescent may suggest drug intoxication, until a history of a previous schizophrenic episode is obtained, and negative laboratory and physical examination data suggest acute schizophrenia as a better bet. The mental status examination must be considered together with the history, physical examination, and laboratory data. An accurate diagnosis requires the synthesis of data from all these sources.

Additional Readings

MacKinnon RA: Psychiatric history and mental status examination, in Comprehensive Textbook of Psychiatry—III. Edited by Freedman AM, Kaplan HI, Sadock BJ. Baltimore, Williams & Wilkins, 1980, Chapter 12.2, pp 906–920

MacKinnon RA, Michels R: The Psychiatric Interview in Clinical Practice. Philadelphia, WB Saunders, 1971

Manschreck TC, Keller MB: The mental status examination: General considerations. The biological mental status examination, in Outpatient Psychiatry Diagnosis and Treatment. Edited by Lazare A. Baltimore, Williams & Wilkins, 1979, Chapters 9, 10, and 11, pp 172–214 (This is a good in-depth discussion of the mental status examination, its validity and reliability)

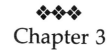

Chapter 3

Psychopathological Processes

Magnus Lakovics

The process of development of psychiatric symptoms and disorders is complex. In the past, it was simpler to study the mind and body separately. Researchers have attempted to explain how the mind works without the benefit of detailed and sometimes even **basic** knowledge of the relationships between neurochemical processes, personality development, thought, and emotional experience. Another problem has been the inherent complexity of doing developmental studies of human beings. Although a generation of animals can be studied within a short time span with good controls, it takes years to study human development, with little or no control over the variables. Because of this, techniques involving cross-sectional, follow-up, and longitudinal perspectives have been used. Predictive studies (which can be essential to establish cause-and-effect relationships) are less common and more difficult.

A most important development has been that instead of artificially dividing human beings into two packages (mind and body), we now see that future fruits will be borne by **understanding the complexity of the human being as a unified bio-psycho-social being.** The fact that we can understand the neurophysiology of thought disorder does not also obviate the importance or significance of understanding its meaning to a patient, its impact on his social functioning, and the relationship of all three with one another.

The literature is filled with attempts to explain disorders from each of these perspectives. Thus, in the course of his psychoanalytic investigations, Sigmund Freud clarified that certain mental content and processes existed outside of awareness (in the *unconscious*); and postulated three theoretical structures or attributes of the mind. These remain useful today to explain the basis of neurotic symptom formation and personality traits. Within this framework, one part (the *id*) consists of our inherent drives, instincts, and physiological needs which, for the most part, are unconscious. Another part is our *ego*. This is the perceiving and regulating part that orders and interprets our behaviors, sensations, and conscious thinking. The third (the *superego*) serves the functions of conscience, and is both conscious and unconscious. This derives from parental and social identifications, and from values incorporated through the process of growing up. As Freud has clarified, neurotic symptom formation results from the difficulty the patient's ego has in managing unpleasant stimuli arising from drives, feelings, and instinctual wishes that are unconscious and not adequately dealt with in the child's early developmental periods because of frustration, overindulgence, or prohibitions arising from an overly strict conscience.

Other theorists (interpersonal and experiential) feel that interpersonal relationships within the culture, social milieu, and the person's here-and-now daily life experience, in and outside the immediate family, is at least as important as the forces identified by Freud. On the other hand, behaviorists emphasize the importance of learning in neurotic symptom formation and suggest that it can be unlearned by appropriate modifications of the immediate antecedents and consequences. Finally, biological psychiatrists identify defective neurochemical physiology to explain psychiatric disturbances.

Each of these schools of thought and research has made major contributions to our understanding of the basis of psychiatric disorders. But separately they are inadequate. Only a combination of explanations which includes psychological, social, and biological factors permits us to understand the basis for the development of psychiatric disorders. In the major mental disorders (schizophrenia, major affective disorders, and organic mental disorders), characterized by disturbances in the basic processes of thought, feeling, behavior and cognition, biological explanations for etiology may be most useful. But we can still use the language of psychoanalysis to understand that these patients have severe ego deficits; and that the individual manifestations of the disorder (e.g., the specific content of a delusion) can be understood best in psychoanalytic or social terms.

A discussion of these processes could take many paths. It could pursue one particular orientation, and describe in great detail the phenomenology and development of psychiatric disorder within it. Based on our current understanding it seems best, however, to combine elements of each in understanding the development of these disorders. (For the text that follows refer to Fig. 1.)

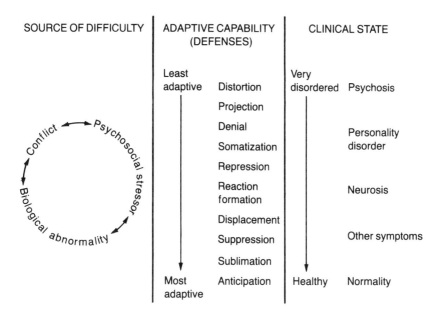

SOURCE OF DIFFICULTY	ADAPTIVE CAPABILITY (DEFENSES)		CLINICAL STATE	
	Least adaptive	Distortion	Very disordered	Psychosis
		Projection		
		Denial		Personality disorder
		Somatization		
		Repression		
		Reaction formation		Neurosis
		Displacement		
		Suppression		Other symptoms
		Sublimation		
	Most adaptive	Anticipation	Healthy	Normality

Figure 1. The psychopathological process.

The source of difficulty in psychiatric disorders can be divided into three basic categories: (1) biological abnormality, (2) intrapsychic conflict, and (3) psychosocial stressors. The term *biological abnormality* refers to changes in the structure or function of the body. *Conflict* is defined as the opposition engendered by simultaneous occurrence of mutually exclusive impulses, desires, or tendencies (e.g., simultaneous feelings of love and hate). The term *psychosocial stressor* refers to life events (including disease) which tend to disrupt the individual's psychological equilibrium. The concepts of *conflict* and *stress* are easily confused. While conflict often arises in the context of life stress, it need not. Moreover, a stressor does not necessarily create conflict. The requirements to perform at a job or school can be stressful because of the demands placed on the person. But he may not feel conflict about this.

Adaptation is a useful concept which can be used to bridge all three categories. This refers to the state of balance between the organism as a whole—the person—and the demands placed on him deriving from both internal and external sources. Under ordinary circumstances, individuals are well adapted. Their adaptive capacity is not exceeded by these demands, that is, they respond to these demands with biological, psychological, and social adjustments which produce minimal disruption in their functioning. Where the demands are excessive in degree and/or the particular individual's adaptive capacities are limited, maladaptation occurs. The maladaptation may involve biological, psychological, and social processes and their complex effects upon one another. It is this complex of effects which we understand as illness, and the signs and symptoms of disorder.

From the psychological standpoint, regardless of the source of difficulty, human beings attempt to adapt by intrapsychic mechanisms called *defenses*. Defenses represent the (unconscious) mental processes which are utilized to adapt to the **meanings** of events of whatever nature. The adaptive capability of human beings depends a great deal on the nature of the particular defenses utilized when confronted by a source of difficulty: biological abnormality, psychological conflict, or life stress. While all defenses are normal, some have only very limited usefulness or are effective only in maintaining intrapsychic balance but are inappropriate (pathological, maladaptive) in dealing with reality. Others are more generally adaptive. In general the degree of effectiveness of a defense in dealing with the demands of reality parallels the developmental sequence in which it develops.

The following is a list of the major psychological defenses, and their definitions, in increasing order of adaptive capability.

Distortion: Reshaping reality to meet one's needs (e.g., feeling entitled to be a professor without the experience and credentials but only because of "superior" knowledge)

Projection: Attributing one's own feelings or wishes to others (e.g., feeling hated by others because of low self-esteem)

Denial: Acting as if a certain reality does not exist (e.g., setting a place at the dinner table for a dead relative)

Somatization (conversion): Conversion of conflict, stress, or problems of living into bodily symptoms

Repression: Deploying an idea, feeling, or conflict out of all conscious awareness

Reaction formation: Adopting a general lifestyle or attitude exactly opposite to the trend of one's actual but unacceptable thoughts and feelings, thereby keeping the latter unconscious (e.g., being overly neat while unconsciously hating it)

Displacement: Shifting the expression of feelings from one person to another person or object that is less dangerous (e.g., being angry at the dog instead of the boss)

Suppression: Intentionally postponing conscious attention to a feeling, wish, etc.

Sublimation: Modifying the natural expression of desire into a socially acceptable form

Anticipation: Planning

In general, the list, beginning with distortion, proceeds from the least generally adaptive defense to the most adaptive, anticipation. This simple generalization is never completely true. In order to demonstrate some of the complexity involved in the adaptive capability of psychological defenses and their relationship to psychiatric disorders, we can use an analogy to physiological homeostasis.

The term *homeostasis* refers to the process whereby the organism maintains all processes within the various limits compatible with sustained life and functioning. When a sufficient demand is placed on one system, other systems (or other parts of the system) are called into play. Changes in those take up the slack, reducing the demand on the system originally taxed. Thus, both function within their adaptive capacities, while the organism remains undamaged and functional. Similarly, defenses function in psychological process to maintain adaptation or psychological equilibrium by responding to the source of difficulty (i.e., demand) through formation of symptoms, character traits, and other action (i.e., output). If a person runs the 100-yard dash, we expect his cardiac output to increase sufficiently to maintain the rapidly utilized oxygen within muscle tissue. If a student is faced with the stress of an examination, he may anticipate the exam and study enough to pass. In the first example, adjustment to increased demand is made by increased cardiac output. In the second, adjustment to the stress on our psychic well-being is made by utilization of a defense we call *anticipation*. In both instances, these are normal mechanisms responding to ordinary demands to maintain adaptation.

Homeostasis and adaptation can be disrupted in two ways: (1) if the stressors are too great for the organism, or (2) if there is some intrinsic abnormality within the organism. With extreme demand, the secondary response itself can become maladaptive, resulting in pathology. With intrinsic abnormalities, maladaptation can occur under conditions of great or even minimal demand.

If the same runner were in a competitive race (high demand) and had not trained sufficiently, his cardiac output and metabolic utilization of oxygen might not be able to meet the need. As a consequence, he might become breathless and be unable to run fast enough. Or if he suffered from a cardiac abnormality he might not even be able to walk normally without disruptive symptoms. Psychological defenses operate similarly. If psychosocial stressors are too great or if a person has a biological abnormality or a developmental defect in psychological maturity, the defenses that attempt to restore well-being may themselves become part of the problem.

Returning to our student, if he suffers not only the stress of the exam, but also learns that he had failed his last exam in his major subject (high demand), he may not be able to adapt effectively and study, but might respond with an attack of severe back pain. The severity of the stressor is great enough to elicit a symptom. Or if he is too immature to utilize anticipation and study, he will have to call on other, less adaptive defenses. In either case he may use the defense of somatization in an attempt to restore intrapsychic well-being, which will create further problems for him. Finally, if the student has had a previous acute schizophrenic episode (presumed biological abnormality), the stress of even a minor exam may make him feel overwhelmed, thereby giving rise to the even more primitive defenses associated with that disorder and resulting in suspiciousness and withdrawal, eventuating in another schizophrenic episode.

Conclusion

An inference may mistakenly be drawn that there is a linear cause-and-effect relationship between the defenses, which are psychological processes, and either the clinical state or the sources of difficulty. This is not intended. The manifestations of a clinical disorder may result from a complex interactive mix of conflict, stressors, and biological abnormality, as well as inappropriate defenses. If a disorder is biologically based, the defective brain structure or function can still operate directly to prevent the utilization of more adaptive defenses, or it can act at an earlier stage of maturation to prevent their formation. Moreover, the impairment itself can add to the demands, calling for more primitive "emergency" defenses. Thus to understand the psychological defenses operating in schizophrenia is not to suggest that the disorder is psychogenic. The converse may also be true. Because a disorder results primarily from intrapsychic conflict and the defenses utilized to cope with that conflict does not mean that biological processes may not be effected.

The concept of *psychological defense* serves many purposes in psychiatry. It is a method of **explaining** the development of some symptoms, a means of **classifying** psychiatric disturbances into diagnostic categories, and also a method of **understanding** a wide range of interpersonal and psychological reactions to sources of difficulty. (Although some psychiatric disorders are classified by the same name as the defenses utilized, most are not. Current classification is based primarily on descriptions of disorders based on categorization of signs and symptoms; or in a few cases—e.g., substance-induced disorder—etiological factors may be used as the basis for a diagnostic category.) Thus, a 59-year-old woman with multiple somatic complaints the onset of which occurred before age 25 may describe herself as being "sickly," and may spend her whole life complaining of loss of sensation, abdominal pains, sexual indifference, and pain in the extremities. She may be **classified as having a somatization disorder;** she may be **understood to use the psycho-**

logical defense of somatization; and she may be observed to **adapt to job stressors with increasing somatization.**

Additional Readings

Hofling CK: Textbook of Psychiatry for Medical Practice. Edited by Hofling CK. Philadelphia, Lippincott, 1975, Chapters 2, 3, 4, pp 25–127 (This is a short, understandable, and readable discussion of psychopathological processes)

Comprehensive Textbook of Psychiatry—III. Edited by Kaplan HI, Freedman AM, Sadock BJ. Baltimore, Williams & Wilkins, 1980

Nemiah JC: The dynamic bases of psychopathology, in The Harvard Guide to Modern Psychiatry. Edited by Nicholi AM. Cambridge, MA, Belknap, 1978, Chapter 9, pp 147–172

Psychopathology: Contributions from the Social, Behavioral and Biological Sciences. Edited by Hamer M, Salzinger K, Sutton A. New York, Wiley, 1973

PART II

PSYCHIATRIC DISORDERS

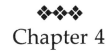

Chapter 4

Organic Brain Syndromes

Donald Oken

The brain is the "organ of the mind." Any disturbance of its neurons, structural or functional, will affect mental functioning. Typically the behavioral effects are general, producing characteristic syndromes which reflect a diffuse impairment in mentation, although relatively isolated defects in mental functions sometimes occur. Because the brain is sensitive to the "internal milieu," systemic disorders commonly give rise to these disturbances, as well as intracranial pathology. Certain causal factors may produce some added specific clinical features. But, **the characteristic clinical syndromes are largely the same, regardless of cause.**

With mental impairment, more primitive behaviors and psychological processes tend to emerge. Consequently, **any psychiatric symptom or sign may appear; and the presenting picture may mimic any other psychiatric disorder.** Thus, organic disorders must be considered in the differential for every psychiatric patient. (George Gershwin entered psychoanalysis only to learn later that he had a brain tumor.) Nevertheless, the characteristic syndrome underlies these presenting symptoms, and can be elicited. This is rarely difficult if the doctor remains alert to this diagnostic possibility, and conducts a thorough mental status examination.

There are two major syndromes: delirium and dementia. *Delirium* is more sudden, transient, dramatic, and related to functional impairment of neurons, typically arising from systemic causes. *Dementia* is more insidious, slowly progressive and enduring, and more often related to neurological disorders. Each presents its particular clinical picture. But the two overlap clinically and in other ways. Delirium may progress into dementia; while patients with even minimal dementia have a very great sensitivity to superimposed delirium. It is essential not to associate this dichotomy with treatability. Many dementias are treatable. Thus, the older parallel terminology of acute vs chronic brain disorders has been discarded because chronic was misinterpreted to mean untreatable.

The diagnostic classification adopted in the new third edition of the Diagnostic and Statistical Manual of Mental Disorders of the American Psychiatric Association (DSM III) includes the "organic brain syndromes" discussed in this chapter as one subcategory of the major category of "organic mental disorders." The other two subcategories are "dementia arising in the senium and presenium," and "substance-induced disorders." The latter, which commonly are due to substances of abuse, including alcohol, have a number of distinctive clinical and physiological features as a group, as well as some related to the specific substance involved. Consequently, these conditions are considered separately (along with problems of abuse per se) in the next chapter, Chapter 5. However, the separation of the senile and presenile dementias is merely etiological, and does not reflect such distinctiveness. Their clinical features are those of the dementias in general; and the information provided in this present chapter applies fully to those conditions.

The clinical manifestations of both delirium and dementia can be understood in terms of basic neurological and psychiatric principles. In general, the sensitivity of neurons to injury parallels the hierarchy of higher to lower brain systems. Most sensitive are the highest, most phylogenetically advanced, developmentally newest centers. These are associated with consciousness and the capacity to acquire new memories and skills and to perform sophisticated intellectual processes.

What is unique to the organic syndromes, and distinguishes them from the other conditions they may mimic, is evidence of this loss of the higher mental functions, revealed in the clinical examination. This is manifest by a **characteristic impairment of the "sensorium," which is diagnostic of these disorders.** These clinical findings, all or some of which may be present, include disturbances in level of consciousness, orientation, perception, memory, and higher cognitive functions: Evidence of these defects is required to make the diagnosis, and is diagnostic in the face of any other psychiatric findings. Abnormalities in the neurological examination may or may not be present.

Anxiety also is common and may be particularly dramatic in delirium. The central reliance which human beings place on their intellectual functions probably is a major reason why that loss is so threatening. An old clinical "pearl" indicates that unexplained monosymptomatic anxiety may be the first clue to the presence of an organic syndrome.

The loss of function of the higher brain centers results in a release of lower centers, just as spasticity occurs in upper-motor-neuron disease. This release results in the escape of primitive impulses, behavior states and emotions, a undermining of prior adjustment, and the substitution of emergency psychological processes. This "regression" is augmented by that due to the aforementioned anxiety. These shifts can produce a presenting clinical picture of any type of severity, with the signs and symptoms of any and every other psychiatric syndrome. One patient may be merely irritable and avoidant, another wildly terrorized by par-

Table I. Common Causes of Organic Brain Syndromes[a]

Metabolic and Endocrine
    Electrolyte imbalances (hyponatremia, etc.)
    Acid–base imbalance
    Dehydration
    Hypo- or hyperglycemia
    Renal failure/azothemia
    Hepatic failure
    Hyper- or hypothyroidism
    Cushing's or Addison's syndrome
Systemic Infections
    Pneumonia
    Pyelonephritis
    Endocarditis
    Any other severe infectious illness
Cardiovascular
    Congestive heart failure
    Acute myocardial infarction
    Pulmonary embolus
Surgery (and anesthesia)
Severe injury (fractures, etc.)
Anoxia
Miscellaneous other systemic illnesses: e.g., acute collagen disease, severe
    hypersensitivity reaction, "acute abdomen"
Intracranial disorders
    Cerebrovascular accidents (stroke) or insufficiency (transient ischemia)
    Tumors (primary or metastatic)
    Trauma: sub- or epidural hemorrhage, contusions, skull fracture
    Infections: acute (meningitis, encephalitis, brain abscess, etc.); chronic (neurosyphilis,
        fungi, tuberculosis, etc.)
    Neurological disorders: multiple sclerosis, Huntington's disease, postictal states,
        epilepsy
    Normal pressure hydrocephalus

[a]In many patients, several of these factors will occur simultaneously. This table omits other types of organic mental disorders which include (1) the syndromes of intoxication, withdrawal, and neuronal damage arising from exogenous drugs; and (2) the dementias arising from Alzheimers or Pick's Disease. The latter, also referred to as senile and presenile dementia, display clinical manifestations no different from dementias due to the above listed causes.

anoid delusions, a third morbidly depressed and suicidal, and a fourth quiet and seemingly normal, all with the same degree of organic impairment. The physician may not simply base his diagnosis on the presenting picture. Unless he searches for evidence of the coexisting underlying defect, he will be misled.

Complete diagnosis is a two-stage process. First, the physician identifies these characteristic clinical findings of impairment on examination. This establishes that there is an organic disorder. Second, additional data are used to establish the specific etiology. In contrast, this almost always comes from the history and/or physical examination. This step is by no means unimportant, for specific etiological diagnosis is key for treatment. But it rests on the initial clinical determination that there is a disorder of the organic type.

The common causes of organic brain syndromes are listed in Table I.

Delirium

The core clinical abnormality in delirium is an impaired level of consciousness. Gross obtundation is obvious, but milder decrements require diagnostic sensitivity. The patient simply may be not quite "with it," a trace foggy or confused. Subjective perplexity and confusion may be reported. Limitations are noted in the patient's ability to focus, shift, or sustain attention; and he may periodically "drift off." Difficulty in sustaining a train of thought leads to a degree of lack of clarity, directiveness, and coherence of speech, which may become disjointed or disorganized. Periods of recent sleepiness or extra naps may be reported. Conversely, anxious hypervigilance may interrupt or prevent normal sleep and produce restlessness; or there may be fluctuation between both extremes.

Perceptual disturbances are very common. Because of the sleeplike alteration of consciousness, there are often reports of unusually vivid and disturbing dreams which the patient cannot clearly differentiate from reality. *Illusions* may occur: distortions of interpretation of real perceptual events, often fearful in content, e.g., interpreting a shadowy fluttering window-curtain at night as an entering intruder until the light is turned on. (These transient tricks of the mind, which occur in normal people, are to be distinguished from *hallucinations*. The latter lack a realistic perceptual basis and are near impossible to correct.) Probably for related reasons, visual hallucinations are not uncommon. (In contrast, the hallucinations of most other disorders are predominantly auditory.)

Disorientation is typical, most notably for time, especially day of week or time of day. Inability to identify place suggests a somewhat more severe disturbance, though it is more likely if the patient recently has been moved (e.g., to the hospital). Disorientation as to one's person occurs only in extreme states.

Disturbance of memory also is common. This is most (or only) evident in a loss of the ability to retain material only very **recently** acquired. The *three-objects test* may be useful in eliciting this: inquiring, after an interval of several minutes, for the names of three items previously listed as being the subject of later inquiry. Care must be taken to have the patient repeat this initially, to ensure that they were heard and registered.

Limitations are seen also in the capacity to recall less immediate, though relatively recent material, particularly of an impersonal nature, such as current events. Similarly, the patient may be unable to specifically identify, or even recognize, people he has seen before, especially if the contact has been recent or infrequent.

The *serial sevens test* is a time-honored device for eliciting the deficit. Requiring attentiveness, concentration, and immediate recall, this requires the patient to subtract by seven repetitively from 100. Unfortunately, this test is more often poorly administered and misinterpreted than otherwise. The key issue is not the accuracy of the calculation, but the capacity of the patient to remember recurrently where he is "at," and to perform the proper task at the time. The sought-for defect is more evident in the type of error and the nature of expressed difficulties than in correctness alone. The usefulness of this test is dependent also on enlisting cooperation, allaying anxiety, and modifying the technique to match IQ and education, e.g., by substituting three or 13 for seven.

Any of the variety of cognitive defects typical of dementia (to be described later) also may occur.

Fluctuation in severity at varying times is characteristic, and may be a clue to diagnosis. Typically, evening and night are the worst times, probably due both to darkness and diurnal shifts in metabolism. But changes even from one hour (or few minutes) to the next are common.

Because anything which impairs brain function can produce delirium, its **causes** are manifold and very common. Any significant disturbance of metabolic or electrolyte function, toxic infections, idiosyncratic drug responses, congestive failure, or other serious illness may produce delirium, as may head injuries, strokes, or neurologic disease. It is likely that delirium occurs in as many as 20% of general hospital patients in the course of their stay. In otherwise unexplained delirium, the most likely cause is some medication.

Sometimes the clinical picture will offer hints as to etiology. Steroids, for example, typically produce affective symptoms, mimicking mania or depression. But these are rarely more than clues, at best. It is the physical examination, history (obtained from family or friends, where necessary), or laboratory tests that provide the major evidence.

Treatment is two-pronged. The basic approach is directed at the

cause(s): either the basic etiology (e.g., antibiotics for infections) or the abnormal pathophysiology (correction of electrolyte disturbances, anoxia, congestive failure, etc.). Because minor associated pathophysiological disturbances may critically tip the balance of cerebral function, additional supportive measures should be directed to correct these. Thus, a patient with pneumonia may benefit greatly from a transfusion for mild anemia, fluids for dehydration, vitamins for borderline nutrition, etc.

Delirium is an acute disorder requiring **active intervention.** The insult to the nervous system may progress rapidly to irreversible neuron damage or even death. Swift, vigorous therapy is important to forestall this. The patient who lies abed quietly obtunded is often in the worst danger, for his undramatic clinical picture may lull physicians and nurses into passivity.

Concomitantly, treatment is directed to the clinical syndrome itself, as dictated by the nature of the disturbance. Excitement, agitation, or disorganization of thought responds to neuroleptics. Barbiturates are contraindicated (except in epileptics). They disrupt neuronal metabolism, and tend to increase delirium. Depression should alert the physician to evaluate suicidal potential and to institute appropriate precautions. Anxiety without these accompaniments will respond to benzodiazepines and to reassurance. The patient should be given simple, brief, concrete explanations about the transient, treatable nature of the disturbance; and immediately relevant, corrective information about orientation or perceptual distortions. Familiarity and stability of the environment are helpful, as is the presence of a recognizable family member. A night-light will reduce the confusion during this time period. Bed-sides, or sometimes restraints, may be required to prevent accidental self-injury. The latter, especially, should be used cautiously, as they may increase fright and agitation.

Dementia

This disorder is characterized by a **deterioration of higher mental functions in the presence of an essentially clear level of consciousness.** A useful screening device for revealing this impairment is the ten-item Brief Mental Status Questionnaire, described on page 135.

Typically, memory is most disturbed. In addition to limitations in the ability to retain immediate information (as in the three-objects test), there are difficulties in recalling past events, especially those in the recent past. The patient's history will have significant gaps and lack specific details which he cannot fill in upon questioning; or he will do so only incompletely and with effort. Less personal and less repetitive events are especially prone to loss (e.g., current events, books, and films).

Knowledge of the weekday and specific date may be lost early. Inability to give the year is more ominous.

Difficulties in performing **calculations** are common, although familiar, simple material, such as multiplication tables, often is retained, as with other old, "overlearned" memories. Defects in the capacity to perform **complex mental tasks** are especially noticeable. The patient may be unable to draw inferences, or see the relationship among those things he does remember or is told. The capacity to deal with **abstract information** is reduced, with overly concrete, simple material substituted. This may be revealed by the patient's interpretation of common proverbs. **Judgment** is likely to be poor. **Personality changes** are common. Preexisting characteristic traits may become exaggerated. Thus, a fussy but effective businessman may become preoccupied with miniscule details, persistently rework fiscal data, and constantly recheck subordinates to the point where office efficiency deteriorates. Or there may be deterioration of prior patterns, and insensitivity to normal social expectations. Unkempt and stained clothing, flirtatiousness, or pedophilia may appear. Mild dyspraxia may be noted, as well as disturbances of subtler coordinated perceptual–motor functions. The latter may be revealed by difficulties in copying three-dimensional figures or complex designs, as in the *Bender Gestalt Test*.

In the full-blown, advanced condition, these and similar difficulties are marked, making the diagnosis apparent. But, typically, dementia begins insidiously. The elicitation and recognition of its subtler early manifestations, already emphasized, are the real task of the physician.

This job is made yet more difficult by the strong tendency of these patients to develop a protective smokescreen: The slow progression allows the patient to develop a variety of defensive, coping, and obscure mechanisms to hide his dreaded impairments, both from himself and others. **These defenses may dominate the presenting clinical picture.** Their presence should alert the physician to this diagnosis, although ultimately (as with delirium) the elicitation of actual cognitive defects is required. By sticking to the familiar, known, concrete, and less complex aspects of the environment, incapacities may be kept hidden. Memory gaps may be covered up by vagueness, perseveration, and shifts of topic. Better remembered, older information may be substituted at distracting length, falsely suggesting that one is dealing merely with the normal tendency of the nondemented aged to focus on the past. Rarely, untrue stories are substituted *(confabulation)*. Partly because "the best defense is a good offense," many patients will be querulous and irritable, driving others away at least from feared topics. This may proceed to the development of a full paranoid picture.

By these devices, and by restricting his activities and constricting his personality, recognition of the mildly demented patient's impairments may be obscured or underestimated for some time. This balance may be shifted suddenly by a change in the patient's life that calls for new learning or more complex adaptations. **Demented patients are extraordinarily sensitive to all types of stressors: biological, psychological, and social.** A move, a new phone number, urban reconstruction or any disruption of personal, social, or family life may produce a sudden decompensation. So can a minimal, transient interference with brain function from a new medication, alcohol, "flu," malnutrition, etc.

This poses a dilemma for the examining physician. The underlying defects must be exposed for diagnosis. Yet too vigorous an exposure results either in heightened defensiveness, upsetting the doctor–patient relationship, or an antitherapeutic decompensation. Considerable tact, gentleness, and sensitivity to the patient's self-respect are required. Impairments must be explored thoroughly, but in a manner that avoids confronting the patient with the implications of his disclosures.

Treatment is similar to that of delirium, with greater emphasis on the correction of all minor contributory physiological abnormalities, and on maintaining or restoring environmental stability. The latter usually requires the involvement of the family, and support to help them cope with the problems posed by the patient.

Other than a failure to make the diagnosis, **the physician's commonest error is undue therapeutic pessimism,** particularly true with the older patient, who may be written off as "just senile." A special instance of this is the misdiagnosis of the pseudodementia which is a common feature of depressive disorders in the aged. But a number of causes of true dementia are correctable: Older people develop brain tumors, subdural hematomas, etc. Also a well-adjusted, mildly demented person may decompensate only because of superimposed, correctable problems. The damaged brain can be exquisitely sensitive to any of the disturbances which cause delirium; and the superimposed delirium may appear merely as progression or decompensation of the dementia. On the psychosocial side, any disruption in the stability of the patient's life or social support system may undermine a stable adjustment: death of a family member, change in living conditions, etc. Often multiple, seemingly minor causes are involved. Treatment must be directed to each.

The second step of the two-part diagnostic process already noted must, therefore, not be neglected in any patient with a newly diagnosed dementia or significant exacerbation. It is necessary to pursue the etiological bases of dementia with greater gentleness in the aged, lest the procedures themselves be added stressors. But no less thoroughness is required. Basic examinations that are least invasive or physiologically disruptive are done first, especially where hospitalization or other moves can be avoided. Usually there is time to allow deliberate pacing. No tests are done without reasonable indication, but all leads are pursued with whatever procedures are required to unravel them. The doctor must remember also that the response to treatment tends to be slow in the aged. Well after correction of the causes, it takes substantial time for the disrupted adaptive capacities to become restored. Patience is called for, along with cautious optimism.

Because of these factors, **whenever there is uncertainty in differentiating delirium from dementia, the former diagnosis alone always should be made,** and appropriate treatment pursued vigorously. Only if it becomes clear later that the full extent of the deficits were chronically preexistant, or that a further acute insult has had new permanent effects, should the diagnosis of dementia be substituted or added.

Additional Considerations

In occasional patients, a single presenting psychiatric symptom dominates the clinical picture, and the generalized impairment characteristic of delirium and dementia is not elicited by the standard mental status examination. Usually, evidence of the characteristic impairment can be found by expert, painstaking reexamination or via special laboratory studies (to be described). These patients may present only with a delusion (organic delusional syndrome), hallucinations (organic hallucinosis), memory disturbance (organic amnestic syndrome), affective symptoms (organic affective syndrome) or personality changes (organic personality syndrome). Clearly, such patients present a difficult diagnostic problem, requiring study by an expert psychiatrist. Nevertheless, usually there are sufficient atypical features to make other diagnoses unsatisfactory and to alert the nonpsychiatrist to the need for such referral. And they are relatively rare.

Two laboratory procedures may be useful in diagnosing the presence of an organic disorder: the electroencephalogram (EEG) and neuropsychological testing.

The normal EEG reveals a predominant waxing–waning pattern of 8 to 12 per second "alpha" waves in most people. Most useful is the bioccipital lead, where alpha usually is most prominent. **In delirium, the predominant EEG rhythm slows.** Where clinical data are suggestive but equivocal, an EEG may resolve the problem. The extent of the slowing is roughly proportional to the degree of cerebral impairment, unlike the severity of the presenting symptoms. Thus, the EEG also can be a useful index of progress. Because a minority of normal people never have alpha, its absence is not absolutely diagnostic unless one knows it was present in a prior EEG; though the presence of a well-developed pattern of slow waves is very suggestive. Also, the EEG is not particularly helpful in dementia, as could be expected from the preservation of normal consciousness. Slowing may be present, but typically this occurs only in advanced cases where no diagnostic problem arises.

In contrast, **neuropsychological tests** have especial diagnostic usefulness for dementia. A variety of special procedures have been developed which have very high sensitivity and specificity. Even the site of a focal lesion may be pinpointed by its characteristic pattern of defects. Also the precise nature of cognitive defects can be identified (e.g., nominal aphasia, visual–motor spacial incoordination), which may suggest more specific and effective rehabilitative measures. Traditional clinical psychological tests also have a significant, though much more limited, value. When dementia is suspected but cannot be confirmed, consultation with a clinical neuropsychologist (or, if unavailable, a general clinical psychologist) is indicated.

Additional Readings

Cummings J, Benson F, LaVerme S: Reversible dementia. JAMA 243:2434–2439, 1980

Diagnostic and Statistical Manual of Mental Disorders, 3rd ed. (DSM III). Washington, DC, American Psychiatric Association, 1980

Engel GL, Romano J: Delirium, A syndrome of cerebral insufficiency. J Chronic Dis 9:260–277, 1959

Goldstein K: Functional disturbances in brain damage, in American Handbook of Psychiatry, 2nd ed, Vol IV. Edited by Arieti S, Reiser MF. New York, Basic Books, 1975

Psychiatric Aspects of Neurological Disease. Edited by Benson DF, Blumer D. New York, Grune & Stratton, 1975

Senility reconsidered: Treatment possibilities for mental impairment in the elderly. Report of the Task Force Sponsored by the National Institute on Aging. JAMA 244:259–263, 1980

Wells CE: Chronic brain disease: An overview. Am J Psychiat 135:1–12, 1978

Wells CE, Duncan GW: Neurology for Psychiatrists. Philadelphia, Davis, 1980, Chapters 3, 5; pp 45–64, 77–96

Chapter 5

Disorders Related to Substance Abuse

Sidney Cohen

It is necessary to routinely consider the effects of drug misuse and abuse in the differential diagnosis of many neuropsychiatric and medical–surgical conditions. Substance abuse or the misuse of prescribed medications rate among the more common of emergency room and hospital admissions. They tend to be complicated cases with multiple disabilities. For example, a comatose patient with a blood alcohol level of 3.5% may also have fallen or been hit on the head, thereby developing an expanding subdural hematoma. Furthermore, problems of multiple use of illicit substances that are routinely adulterated, misbranded and without any quality control, also complicates the clinical picture.

For each of the drugs or drug classes under discussion the diagnosis and management of the intoxicated state, the overdose syndrome, the withdrawal symptomatology, and certain special complications will be described. It is not possible to be exhaustive here, but expanded discussions of the important issues will be found at the end of this chapter under Additional Readings.

The abuse of chemicals can mimic many other psychiatric disorders. Hallucinogens, amphetamines, and phencyclidine (PCP) can present with a picture that closely resembles acute paranoid schizophrenia. Urine screens for these drugs may be needed to clarify the diagnosis. Even the toxic psychosis caused by anticholinergic drugs may be mistaken for a florid endogenous psychosis. Anxiety, depression, and other mood, thought, and behavioral disorders might be the result of, as well as the cause of, excessive drug taking. Those individuals in psychological distress are more likely to be overinvolved in consciousness-changing chemicals. They attempt to self-treat their dysphoria, and the temporary relief obtained establishes the drug-using career.

Central Nervous System Depressants

Hypnosedatives

This class includes the sleeping medications, and the daytime sedatives (minor tranquilizers, anxiolytics). The **barbiturates and the benzodiazepines** are the principal subgroups. Although important differences between them exist, the intoxicated, overdose, and withdrawal states are rather similar. **These states also resemble that induced by alcohol,** and cross-tolerance and synergistic effects between ethanol and the hypnosedatives occur.

INTOXICATION

After a preliminary phase of disinhibited behavior, progressive depression of the cortical and subcortical functions take place. Euphoria, later dysphoria, impaired memory, judgment, psychomotor dexterity, and varying degrees of confusion can develop. Neurological symptoms include: slurred speech, ataxia, and lateral nystagmus. Irascibility, violent acting out, and accident proneness are not uncommon. Drowsiness or stupor are frequently seen. Reflexes are depressed except during methaqualone (Quaalude) intoxication, when they are usually hyperactive. These drugs can be detected in blood and urine.

OVERDOSE

Coma with severely depressed respirations and blood pressure, normal or slightly contracted pupils (except with hypoxia or glutethimide—Doriden—overdose, when they are dilated) are the signs of overdose. The patient may be in shock. **Delirium** rather than coma may be present. Tachycardia, hemoconcentration, hypothermia, and respiratory acidosis are to be anticipated. Skin bullae on the pressure-bearing areas are seen in protracted comatose states.

The ratio of the lethal to the therapeutic dose of the barbiturates is about 12:1 in a nontolerant person. For the benzodiazepines it is more than 100:1. Combinations of CNS depressants are at least additive in their effects. The combined use of barbiturates and alcohol is supraadditive due to competition for the available hepatic endoplasmic reticular enzymes.

WITHDRAWAL

After tolerance has developed to five or more average daily doses of some hypnosedative, their abrupt discontinuance leads to the fairly consistent symptomatology of the abstinence syndrome. It is **identical to** the alcoholic **delirium tremens (DTs),** and its intensity varies depending upon the amount and duration of the excessive sedative–hypnotic use. The early symptoms consist of a coarse tremor, insomnia, nausea, fever, anxiety, and orthostatic hypotension. Later, the patient may develop a toxic psychosis (delirium) with visual illusions of hallucinations, agitation, and poor attention span. One or a series of grand mal convulsions may intervene after the second or third day.

TREATMENT

The management of **intoxication** may require only close observation of the patient and the vital signs to be assured that he is protected, and that the condition is not progressively worsening. Gastric lavage or induced emesis might be considered if the drug has been taken less than 4 hours previously. The **overdosed, comatose** patient with embarrassed respiratory function requires a patent airway, oxygen, assisted respirations if apnea is present, and the management of cardiovascular collapse. Intravenous lines, parenteral fluids, vasopressors, antibiotics, and an indwelling urethral catheter are often indicated.

Intravenous diazepam (Valium) 10 mg or phenytoin (Dilantin) 600 mg are a satisfactory preventive or treatment for convulsions. Blood chemistries, blood counts, blood gases, urine analysis, EKGs, chest and perhaps other x-rays will be required for additional diagnosis and to observe the course of treatment. The vital signs must be frequently monitored. **Analeptics have no role** in coma due to depressant drugs.

When a suicide attempt was the reason for the overdose, referral for psychiatric evaluation and care will be indicated. If the intoxication or overdose resulted from drug dependence, a referral to a drug abuse clinic or the patient's private physician is worthwhile. If a physician assumes responsibility for the treatment of a drug-dependent patient, he must be aware of the possibility that bids for psychotropic drugs will be made. These must be carefully evaluated and openly dealt with.

The patient in hypnosedative **withdrawal** requires a gradual reduction of that drug or some agent that has cross-tolerance with it. Secobarbital or phenobarbital are commonly used for detoxification from barbiturates or other sedative nonbenzodiazepines. For alcohol and benzodiazepine withdrawal states, chlordiazepoxide or diazepam has been most commonly employed. When the quantity of chronic sedative use is known, the safest procedure is to stabilize on the previous daily dosage. Otherwise, treatment can be started with 200 mg of secobarbital. In 2 hours the patient should be reexamined. If mild intoxication is present (slightly slurred speech, swaying but not falling on the Romberg test, nystagmus) the dose can be repeated. If the patient is asleep or definitely intoxicated, the dose is omitted. If withdrawal symptoms are present (tremulousness, agitation, twitching) 300 mg of secobarbital should be given. This procedure is repeated every 2 hours. The total 24-hour dose can then be calculated and given in four daily doses. A reduction of 100 mg a day thereafter is safe. Instead of each 100-mg dose of a rapid-acting barbiturate, 30 mg of phenobarbital can be substituted. It has the advantage of producing a more stable blood barbiturate level.

Alcohol

As mentioned above, the intoxicated, overdosed, and withdrawal states due to alcohol are similar to that of the hypnosedatives, and their management is similar. The odor of ethanol is, of course, distinctive, but **the diagnostic search should not end after ethanol intake has been established.** Polydrug use and many other causes of delirium, coma, and convulsions must be considered.

INTOXICATION

Simple intoxication is traditionally treated by oneself or those in touch with the drunken individual. Severe intoxication and coma are life-threatening only when the person is debilitated or suffers from one of the complications such as pneumonia, atelectasis, major trauma, concurrent diabetic coma, or severe head injury.

It is **dysfunctional behavior** while intoxicated that accounts for much of the morbidity and mortality associated with ethanol. Fatal accidents, homicides, suicides, battered children and spouses, rape, and other aggressive acts make this drug the most destructive of all. Assaultiveness is particularly notable under conditions of **pathological intoxication** in which small amounts of alcohol produce loss of controls over behavior; such instances are often related to previous head injury.

OVERDOSE

Death from overdose of alcohol-containing beverages alone is infrequent. A built-in safeguard exists in that coma intervenes before a lethal amount can be swallowed unless a very large quantity is ingested within a few minutes. Accidental or suicidal overdose ordinarily results from combinations of alcohol with other depressant drugs.

WITHDRAWAL

In addition to the DTs, as described under hypnosedative withdrawal, other abstinence syndromes are seen. The hangover is considered a manifestation of early withdrawal by some investigators. The impending DTs consist of anxiety, tremulousness, and mild clouding of the sensorium. This is to be distinguished from acute alcoholic hallucinosis, which is notable in that auditory hallucinations occur in the absence of confusion or other symptoms of withdrawal. Impending DTs also must be differentiated from a schizophrenic reaction.

NUTRITIONAL DISORDERS

A group of nutritional disorders are associated with chronic alcoholism and malnutrition and often appear following the postwithdrawal state. The neuropsychiatric syndromes include:

Wernicke–Korsakoff Encephalopathy, of which polyneuritis, ataxia, ocular palsies, ptosis, and dementia with confabulation are frequent signs. A specific thiamine deficiency is responsible.

Cerebellar degeneration, in which gait and trunk ataxia are apparent.

Amblyopia, which is usually found in heavy tobacco and alcohol users.

Cerebral degeneration, in which progressive alcoholic dementia, astasia–abasia, and retropulsion occur due to widespread demyelinization of the cortex.

Marchiafava–Bignami disease, which consists of demyelination of the corpus collosum and presents with a progressive dementia.

Pellagra–niacin deficiency, which causes dermatitis, diarrhea, and dementia.

Central pontine myelinolysis, which is rare, and is manifested by dysphagia and dysarthria.

TREATMENT

Acutely **intoxicated** patients should be protected from injuring themselves or others. Fructose has not been proven to be more effective than glucose in decreasing blood alcohol complications, and may induce hyperuricemia or lactic acidosis.

Lethal **overdose** has occurred at blood alcohol concentrations of 350 mg/dl in nontolerant individuals, while tolerant imbibers have survived levels of 450 to 500 mg/dl. Support of vital functions and a search for complicating injuries, infections and diseases are the principles of therapy. **Withdrawal** is generally carried out with decreasing doses of chlordiazepoxide, multivitamins (including large doses of thiamine), and the correction of electrolyte abnormalities. Sleep and rest are essential, and general nutritional, nursing, and psychological supportive measures are important aspects of treatment. Propylactin anticonvulsant medication may be required.

It is not the end stages of organic brain disease noted above that constitutes the major problem. Instead, it is the much larger number of partially impaired alcoholics whose mentation is blunted, and who have little insight into their rehabilitation.

After recovery, the problem of excessive drinking remains, and the **long-term therapy of problem drinking** begins. It is rare that alcohol abusers will change their drinking patterns, even after shattering experiences with the DTs or life-threatening injuries or illnesses due to their drinking. Combinations of individual, family or group counseling, behavior modification, Alcoholics Anonymous, and disulfiram are among the more common therapies employed.

Narcotics

The narcotics are either opium alkaloids (morphine), opium derivatives (heroin), or synthetics (methadone) that act as analgesics, hypnotics, and drive reducers. They occupy endorphin receptor sites in the CNS and elsewhere. Cross-tolerance between members of this class exists. Dependence evolves from occasional to daily usage. After a week or more of multiple daily doses, the abstinence syndrome appears upon sudden withdrawal.

INTOXICATION

If the opioid is taken intravenously by someone who is addicted, the sought-after effects are a brief, orgasmic euphoria fading in an hour or two into a warm, pleasant, dreamy state (nodding). This is followed by a period of normal or increased activity accompanied by a sense of well-being that later wanes and is replaced by irritability and a compelling desire to return to the narcotized state.

Pupillary constriction, drowsiness, and a general diminution of awareness and mental acuity are characteristic of the intoxicated state. Constipation, and loss of interest in food and sexual activity are frequent complaints of regular users. The skin complications of multiple, less-than-sterile injections are seen in more chronic users.

OVERDOSE

The pupils are pinpoint and nonreactive. Respirations are depressed or absent, and cyanosis and pulmonary edema may be present. Hypotension with shock, hypothermia, and tachycardia are commonly found. The patient may be stuporous or deeply comatose. Reflexes are diminished or unobtainable. The classical triad of pinpoint pupils, depressed respiration, and coma is a hallmark of opioid overdose. However, when anoxia is severe, the pupils may dilate. Meperidine (Demerol) can cause convulsions.

Opiates are readily found in the urine, but a more elegant test is the use of 0.4 mg of naloxone intravenously. Within 2 minutes the coma, respiratory depression, and miosis will be partly or completely reversed.

WITHDRAWAL

The abrupt discontinuance from substantial opiate use results in **the release of adrenergic activity** that had been suppressed. Currently the abstinence syndrome usually presents with moderate discomfort, irritability, and demands for opiates. But the full-blown picture of withdrawal from large amounts of relatively pure material is still sometimes seen. These mimic a very severe case of the flu. Rhinorrhea, lacrimation, diarrhea, pupillary dilation, and sweating occur. Fever, muscle aches, and spasms ("kicking the habit") are seen. Pilorection is an objective sign of withdrawal. Insomnia or a fitful sleep will be present along with nausea, anorexia, and vomiting. Yawning respirations and tachycardia are ordinarily noted.

Injections of naloxone (Narcan) or nalorphine (Nalline) can induce withdrawal in a person who has been using full doses of an opioid for more than a week. In small amounts these narcotic antagonists can be used as a diagnostic test for recent opiate usage. They will produce pupillary dilation, reversing the contracted pupils.

COMPLICATIONS OF CHRONIC DEPENDENCE

Aside from overdose, analphylactic reactions to the adulterants in street heroin and withdrawal, the complications of heroinism are those of unsterility. Hepatitis is almost invariable during a career of heroin addiction. Thrombophlebitis, blood stream infections, endocarditis, and a variety of forms of cellulitis are consistently reported. Tetanus is more likely to occur in female addicts because they tend to "skin pop" more than men and are less likely to have been immunized with tetanus toxoid. The presence of quinine as an adulterant may also predispose to the anaerobic growth of *C. tetani*. Malaria is an infrequently transmitted infection. Metastatic abscesses of any organ, including the brain, might be detected. Pneumonia from aspiration while comatose and pulmonary edema due to the severe depression of the respiratory center are not infrequently found.

Neonatal abstinence symptoms can be encountered with mothers using heroin or on methadone maintenance. The presenting signs are a flapping tremor, tachypnea, yawning, muscle jerks, and convulsive episodes. These should be treated with decreasing doses of paragoric or methadone.

TREATMENT

Active treatment of opioid **intoxication** may not be necessary if vital signs are unaffected, and the patient is drowsy or sleeping. For an actual **overdose, two procedures are immediately necessary.** One is the intravenous use of naloxone 0.4 mg, repeated as necessary every quarter-hour; and the second is the establishment of a patent airway with ventilatory assistance. **The narcotic antagonist will be of no value in non-opioid coma; neither will it be harmful.** Of course, shock and pulmonary edema will require treatment if they are present.

In mild opiate "habits" the patient may need little assistance during

withdrawal. Sedatives and anticholinergic drugs may be sufficient. When obvious withdrawal effects are present, it is customary to gradually detoxify with 20 to 40 mg of methadone orally. This initial dose is reduced by 5 mg daily. On this program the patient should be relatively comfortable, although complaints are to be expected. The alpha-adrenergic agonist clonidine (Catapress) has recently been found effective in opiate withdrawal.

Following detoxification from opioids the **reeducation and rehabilitation** of the addicted individual is required. *Therapeutic communities* are live-in groups that employ reinforcing techniques to promote the development and perpetuation of abstinent behavior. Maintenance with methadone is another therapeutic device that provides oral, single daily doses of methadone (20 to 120 mg). Opiate craving is reduced, and injected heroin has little or no effect, due to cross-tolerance. Methadone maintenance should be combined with counseling and other ancillary aids like vocational rehabilitation. These latter procedures may, in themselves, be sufficient to ensure abstinence. Narcotic antagonists have been employed therapeutically to block opiate effects and thereby assure an opiate-free existence.

The law forbids the private physician to maintain addicts on narcotic drugs except when hospitalized for medical, surgical, or obstetrical problems. **Prescription blank security** is a continuing requirement when dealing with drug-dependent patients. Learning the "conning" techniques of such persons is necessary.

Methadone maintenance patients requiring hospitalization for medical or surgical reasons should not have their methadone dosage altered except with the concurrence of the drug treatment physician. Average doses of other opiates will provide analgesia if that is needed. Pentazocine (Talwin) should not be used because it is a partial narcotic antagonist.

Street addicts on unknown amounts of heroin who are admitted to a hospital for some medical or surgical condition should be placed on 5 to 20 mg of methadone orally daily, depending upon the severity of their opiate withdrawal. A total of 30 mg of methadone a day, or less, is generally ample to keep the patient relatively comfortable during the acute phase of the illness.

Volatile Solvents

The industrial inhalants (toluene, acetone, xylene, methyl ethyl ketone, etc.) when inhaled produce an inebriated state similar to alcohol except that it comes on more rapidly and is briefer. Overdose states are not frequently seen. Withdrawal symptoms, except for irritability, are rarely described. When death occurs, it is due to cardiac asystole from the effect of the solvent on a hypoxic myocardium.

The problems of management are essentially those of dealing with an adolescent polydrug pattern of behavior. Peer group counseling and behavior modification procedures are worth trying. As with alcoholism, solventism can be associated with neuropsychological dysfunction during the sober interval that makes cognitive therapies difficult and motivation less than optimal.

Cannabis (Marijuana)

Although marijuana and its active ingredient, delta-9-THC, belong in the hallucinogenic class of drugs, its depressant effects require placing it in the CNS-depressant category. Simple intoxication requires no intervention except in those rare instances when panic or paranoid reactions occur. It is accompanied by injection of the conjunctiva (red eye) and tachycardia. The mental condition is one of relaxation and a dreamy, reverie state. Overdose is extremely rare, and is characterized by hallucinatory and delusional experiences. Tolerance develops when large amounts are consumed or smoked consistently, but the withdrawal syndrome consists only of minor symptoms like restlessness, nausea, anorexia, and insomnia. The question of amotivation in heavy users remains unresolved.

Treatment may be required in connection with persistent, heavy use, especially in juveniles. Conventional psychotherapies have been occasionally successful. Substitution of alternative behaviors, for example, meditation, has met with some success. The physician is often called on by parents for advice about the cannabis use of their child.

Anticholinergic Drugs

Occasional outbreaks of adolescent use of certain wild plants and medications can produce a picture of atropine poisoning. In this country jimsonweed *(Datura strammonuim)* is the most common weed that intoxicates accidentally or deliberately. Belladonna, henbane, and angel's trumpet have also been involved. In addition, drugs used for Parkinsonism, like trihexyphenidyl (Artane), have been sporadically used in excess to induce a delirium. Tricyclic antidepressants like amytriptyline (Elavil) have an occasional popularity, due to their anticholinergic and sedative qualities.

The **symptoms** are distinctive: red face, dry skin and mucous membranes, maximally dilated pupils, picking movement and a confused muttering, delirium, or coma. Overdose can persist for days if untreated because the gastrointestinal tract is paralyzed and absorption continues.

Treatment, in addition to gastric lavage, consists of intravenous physostigmine 1 or 2 mg given slowly. This should reverse most of the symptoms noted above. It may be necessary to repeat the injection at intervals.

Central Nervous System Stimulants

As a class, these agents produce low-voltage, fast-wave activation of the EEG. Many have some therapeutic usefulness as anorectics, in the treatment of juvenile hyperkinetic behavioral disorders, and for narcolepsy. They act by releasing norepinephrine into the synaptic cleft, preventing its reuptake, and stimulating either alpha- or beta-adrenergic receptors, or both.

Amphetamines and Related Compounds

INTOXICATION

Intoxication with drugs of the amphetamine group includes dilated, reactive pupils, elevated blood pressure and heart rate, hyperactive deep reflexes, dry mouth, sweating, a fine tremor, and loss of appetite. Overactivity, loquacity, jitteriness, impulsivity, and insomnia are often present. Euphoria is frequent, but dysphoria is also seen. Hypervigilance, mild confusion, and impaired judgment are possible consequences.

OVERDOSE

Amphetamine-type poisoning consists of a variety of states. **Paranoid psychoses** resembling schizophrenia, and **unpredictable aggressiveness** are possibilities. Cerebral hemorrhage from the paroxysmal hypertension has been reported, as has cardiac arrhythmias. Stereotyped behaviors and markedly impaired judgment are seen in high-dose states. Amphetamine overdose culminates in hyperpyrexia, convulsions, and coma. **A urine screen can confirm the diagnosis.**

WITHDRAWAL

After tolerance has developed, a stimulant withdrawal syndrome can be identified. It consists of lethargy and hypersomnia, a ravenous appetite, multiple muscle aches and pains, fatigue, and a prolonged psychic depression of varying intensity.

TREATMENT

The physiological antidote for the amphetamine-type drugs is the **antipsychotic agents,** such as chlorpromazine or haloperidol. Barbiturates can also be used in instances of intoxicated behavior requiring modulation. The high fever that accompanies overdose may require cooling measures. Convulsions can be treated with intravenous diazepam 10 mg given intravenously slowly. Hypertensive crises are managed with an intravenous antihypertensive agent. Acidification of the urine with ascorbic acid, cranberry juice, or ammonium chloride increases amphetamine excretion rates.

Withdrawal, even from high doses of amphetamines, can be accomplished abruptly. This may be stressful, and gradual withdrawal is sometimes practiced in hospital situations. Tricyclic antidepressants are indicated in serious depressive reactions. Mild analgesics for achiness, and nutritional supplementation for malnutrition may be required. If the paranoid psychotic reaction persists, the neuroleptics should be used.

Cocaine

Cocaine can be conceptualized as a rapid-acting, short-lasting amphetamine. Its brevity of action can be measured in minutes, and it therefore evades some of the toxic effects of the amphetamines. However, paranoid states resembling the amphetamine schizophreniform psychosis can develop with sustained usage. The intravenous or smoked mode of use is more likely to produce adverse effects than the nasal route.

INTOXICATION

Psychic stimulation, elation, even ecstatic moods can be experienced. Increased energy, talkativeness, and feelings of power and confidence are reported by the user. Sometimes excitement, feverishness, and a fine tremor are present.

OVERDOSE

Extreme agitation, suspiciousness, and paranoid breaks with reality are signs of early overdose. Violent behavior, cardiac irregularities, convulsions, and panic states are possible.

WITHDRAWAL

A true withdrawal syndrome does not occur except when enormous amounts are used. What is not infrequent is postcocaine lethargy, asthenia, and depression (the "coke blues").

TREATMENT

Intoxication is usually over before a person presents himself to a medical facility. **Overdose** is managed with intravenous barbiturates, benzodiazepines, or neuroleptics. Cardiorespiratory support may be needed. Hyperpyrexia can be treated with icepacks or an ice mattress.

Caffeine

Caffeine is a widely used drug that produces few adverse effects except in those sensitive to it, or in those who consume large amounts daily. Headache, jitteriness, and anxiety have been noted in such individuals.

Abrupt stoppage of large amounts may result in sluggishness and fatigue for a few days.

Hallucinogens (LSD, etc.)

These are generally CNS stimulants that intensify perception, produce illusions, pseudohallucinations, and less frequently, hallucinations. Thought patterns, self-image, affect, and perception are altered in the direction of right hemispheric dominance. LSD will be used as the prototype of this class.

INTOXICATION

The hallmark of the intoxicated state is chromatic visual displays which are more vivid with closed eyes. Synesthesias, prolongation of the afterimage, slowing of time perception, dissolution of ego boundaries, and depersonalization have all been experienced. The dominant mood is euphoria or elation, but anxiety, panic, or depression are possible. Thinking is nonlinear, and delusional ideas with a paranoid flavor occur. The face is flushed, pupils widely dilated, and deep reflexes hyperactive. Body temperature is elevated, with lesser elevations of blood pressure and pulse rate. The state lasts from 6 to 24 hours, depending on the dose, and is seen by the clinician only when severe dysphoria or acting out of delusional ideas take place.

OVERDOSE

Death from overdose is exceedingly rare. Deaths have been reported from accidents and suicide. The overdose state may be accompanied by convulsions and hyperpyrexia.

WITHDRAWAL

Although tolerance develops rapidly, and cross-tolerance between LSD, mescaline, and psilocybin occurs, a withdrawal syndrome has not been described.

TREATMENT

The most common medical emergency is the **anxiety–panic reaction.** This should be treated with reassurance and support. If medication is necessary, the benzodiazepines are satisfactory. Since the patient is hypersuggestible, hospital routines should be attenuated, and calm observation in a friendly, supportive environment is substituted. The second most common complication is the prolonged psychotic reaction which requires neuroleptics. Flashbacks need reassurance that they will recede over time. Following any of these reactions, management consists of improvement of general health, reduction of stressful activities, and avoidance of all psychotropic drugs, including cannabis and antihistamines.

Phencyclidine (PCP)

PCP is a difficult drug to classify; it has been called both a dissociative anesthetic and an hallucinogen with cerebellar, autonomic, analgesic, anesthetic, and convulsive features. It is capable of producing serious overdose symptoms: delirium, schizophreniclike paranoid psychosis, intense depersonalization, euphoria, depression, spectacular violence, and demonstrations of unusual strength. Vertical nystagmus is a sign almost unique to PCP and ketamine (a related compound) intoxication. Tolerance but no withdrawal effects have been reported.

Treatment of the overdose state includes continuous gastric suction, acidification of the urine with ammonium chloride, administration of diuretics and anticonvulsants, and control of the patient. PCP is alkaline and is reabsorbed into the stomach or excreted readily into an acid urine by ion exchange. The psychotic state may be prolonged and requires neuroleptics. A serious depression may emerge after recovery from the psychotic reaction.

Comments

As one reflects that some 10 million people have alcohol-related problems, a half-million are heroin-dependent, and very large numbers employ the other drugs mentioned here in ways detrimental to their well-being, the magnitude of the problem becomes apparent.

Current trends indicate that the use of multiple drugs together or sequentially complicate an already complex picture. Nor do projections of prevalence indicate that destructive substance abuse is diminishing. It is becoming institutionalized so that media coverage may be diminishing while the consequences of destructive drug use continue to increase.

As indicated, many disorders related to the drugs of abuse resemble neuropsychiatric states like psychosis, dementia, and the affective disorders. Therefore, they must be considered in their differential diagnosis.

Additional Readings

Clark WG, Del Guidice J: Principles of Psychopharmacology. New York, Academic, 1980

Cohen S: The Drug Dilemma. New York, McGraw-Hill, 1976

Dupont RL, Goldstein A, O'Donnell J: Handbook on Drug Abuse. U.S. Government Printing Office, Washington DC, 1979

Goodman LS, Gilman A: The Pharmacological Basis of Therapeutics, 6th ed. New York, Macmillan, 1980

Jarvik ME: Psychopharmacology in the Practice of Medicine. New York, Appleton-Century-Crofts, 1977

Pradhan SN, Dutta SN: Drug Abuse: Clinical and Basic Aspects. St. Louis, Mosby, 1977

Schecter A: Treatment Aspects of Drug Dependence. West Palm Beach, FL, CRC Press, 1978

Chapter 6

Schizophrenic and Paranoid Disorders

Robert Cancro

Approximately 25% of all hospital beds, and approximately one-half of the psychiatric beds in the United States, are occupied by people who carry the diagnosis of a schizophrenic disorder. The lifetime risk of developing such an illness is approximately 1%. The population on whom this diagnosis has been made worldwide is estimated at 10 million. Clearly, the problem presented by this group of disorders is of major proportions both in terms of individual suffering and public health considerations.

Definition of the Schizophrenic Disorder

The understanding of schizophrenia has varied over time and as a function of fashion. It has been conceptualized as everything from a disease of the brain to an alternative lifestyle. The paucity of reliable information available as to its etio–pathogenesis has led to a broad range of often contradictory positions. Nevertheless, it is possible to state a general framework within which the clinician can work effectively to diagnose and treat these disorders.

The schizophrenias represent a group of illnesses whose clinical features, while variable, can be characterized. The origin of these illnesses is unknown; though there are good reasons to assume that biological, psychological, and social components are involved. Thus this group of disorders represents **a syndrome** rather than a disease entity; this term referring to a condition with a relatively consistent pattern of clinical signs and symptoms which may arise from a number of different initial conditions operating through different mechanisms utilizing different pathways. This biological heterogeneity is inherent and not a function of limitations in existing diagnostic methods. It follows logically that the schizophrenic syndrome represents a heterogeneous group of illnesses which share certain features in common, to differing degrees. Because there is no biological test for the schizophrenic syndrome, it is more heterogeneous than a biochemical syndrome such as diabetes mellitus. The diagnostic criteria are entirely clinical in nature, and therefore arbitrary. This lack of independent validation of the diagnosis leads to a second major source of variation in the people so labeled. Ultimately no truly scientific definition and classfication of the schizophrenias can be achieved until there is an adequate taxonomy of its bio-psycho-social origins.

Diagnosis

The major features of these disorders can be specified in terms of a series of **diagnostic criteria,** which include age of onset, disorganization of prior level of functioning, and a tendency towards chronicity—though often these are one or more episodes of acute illness, as well as characteristic symptoms. In addition, certain other psychiatric conditions which may mimic the disorder must be excluded (ruled out). These criteria have been embodied in the current official diagnostic schema of psychiatric disorders, the third edition of the *Diagnostic and Statistical Manual* of the American Psychiatric Association (DSM III).

Age of Onset

Most commonly the disorder aries in late adolescence or early adulthood. Except in rare instances, the diagnosis is not made unless the illness began before age 45.

Chronicity

Clinical experience has indicated that the diagnosis should be reserved for illnesses of **at least 6 months duration, overall.**

For many years, it was common in the United States to use the diagnosis "acute schizophrenia" for relatively brief illnesses manifesting the characteristic symptoms of the active phase of schizophrenia, often in florid form. This proved to have several disadvantages; and that diagnostic term has been dropped. For many of these patients, the subsequent clinical course differed greatly: they recovered quickly and displayed no subsequent evidence of the disorder. Yet, having been given this diagnosis, they suffered both social stigma and undue persistent concerns about their futures (prognosis). And their inclusion as schizophrenia led to a lack of comparability with patients given this diagnosis in other countries, greatly confusing the interpretation of clinical studies. Thus it has proved wiser to use the diagnosis *Schizophreniform Disorders* for patients ill less than 6 months, though otherwise meeting the diagnostic criteria. Some later turn out to have a more persistent illness; and the diagnosis is then corrected (at the 6-month point) to that of Schizophrenic Disorder.

For yet another small subgroup whose schizophreniclike illnesses are even briefer (under 2 weeks) and follow an overt major life stress, the term *Brief Reactive Psychosis* is used. In very rare instances only will these patients later turn out to have a schizophrenic disorder.

While there must be an **active phase** at some point to make the diagnosis, it should be emphasized that this alone need not be present for 6 months or more. There may be prior prodromal phase and/or a subsequent residual phase; and it is the total duration of these that must be of 6 months duration.

Prodromal Phase

Typically the disorder is ushered in by prodromal symptoms, although manifestations of the active phase sometimes occur without these. It is not always easy to identify the precise beginning of the prodromal phase but it is best defined as a clear deterioration of function prior to the active phase, which involves the presence of certain selected symptoms. The recognition of a true prodromal phase may be clarified by the following clinical examples:

CASE 1: A 21-year-old college student began to show increasing disinterest in his school work following the breakup of a romance. He spent much time in bed sleeping, missed classes, and did not study for examinations. He spent very little time with his friends, who were worried about his social withdrawal. He was somewhat neglectful of his personal appearance and did not shave for several days at a time. He was very preoccupied about himself and his value as a person. When the student was seen in the student health service, the psychiatrist could find no delusions, hallucinations, or evidence of psychotic thinking. There was no history of substance abuse, and the patient appeared to be reacting to the loss of his girlfriend with a depressive disorder. The psychiatrist recommended a brief leave of absence from school, and psychotherapy. Within the next few months, the depressive symptoms improved, and by the following semester the student was able to return to school and continue his education successfully. Thus this illness was not the prodromal phase of schizophrenia.

CASE 2: Another 21-year-old college student also began to show significant impairment in his college work following the breakup of a romance. He spent much time in his room reading the Bible. His friends were worried because of his increasing withdrawal and by his neglect of his personal appearance. When he was seen in the student health service, there were no clear-cut psychotic symptoms found on mental status examination, and the patient had no history of substance abuse. He indicated that he read the Bible to seek guidance as to how he should lead his life, despite his previous lack of interest in religious matters. The patient had a vague idea that there was a reason his relationship with his girlfriend had been terminated, but that reason was not yet clear to him. He had vague feelings that perhaps people were talking about him or laughing at him, but this was not absolutely certain in his mind.

The psychiatrist recommended a leave of absence and psychotherapy. Over the next 2 months, the symptoms became increasingly severe, with the development of clear delusions of both a grandiose and religious nature. The patient began to have auditory hallucinations in which the voices commented on his behavior and talked to each other about him. At this time, the diagnosis of a schizophrenic disorder was made.

As is clear from the above, the recognition of the prodromal nature of a particular symptom complex often can only be made after a period of time has elapsed. If no active stage of a schizophrenic psychosis develops, the illness, by definition, was not prodromal.

Prodromal symptoms include social isolation or withdrawal; marked impairment of role functioning; very peculiar behavior; poor grooming or personal hygiene; blunted, flat, or inappropriate affect; unusual perceptual experiences; odd or bizarre ideation or "magical thinking", and digressive, vague, circumstantial, or metaphorical speech. The diagnosis is not made ordinarily unless at least two of these are present.

Active Phase

This is recognized by the presence of certain characteristic symptoms combined with gross impairment in routine everyday functioning. Examples of the latter include work, school, social relations, personal hygiene, and self-care.

Characteristic symptoms include delusions, hallucinations, and disorganization of thought and verbal behavior. These may be of a variety of types. But they are not dependably diagnostic unless two or more are present in addition to disruption of at least two areas of routine functioning.

The typical **delusions** are bizarre, religious, somatic, grandiose, nihilistic, or persecutory—the last being truly characteristic only if accompanied by hallucinations. Characteristic **auditory hallucinations** are those in which two voices converse, or one voice provides running commentary on the patient's behavior, or are repetitive but unrelated to a depressed or elated mood. The typical **thought disturbance** is evident by incoherence, loose associations, illogicality, or poverty of content; but this is not dependable unless accompanied by a flat, blunted, or inappropriate affect, grossly disorganized behavior, or some type of hallucinations or delusions.

Other very common, though not specifically diagnostic symptoms include a disturbed sense of self; "autistic" preoccupation with one's own thoughts and viewpoint; difficulty in making decisions and carrying them out in goal-directed activity; subjective perplexity and confusion; ritualistic behavior, ideas of reference; and dysphoric mood states.

A clinical example may be useful.

CASE 3: A 26-year-old male was brought to an emergency room complaining of people being able to read his mind. He described people on the street knowing what he was thinking in advance of his actually thinking it. He complained that there were individuals who could control his thoughts and put ideas into his head. At times he heard several voices talking to each other and even arguing. He was convinced that he had a special religious mission which involved saving the world from catastrophe. Despite the strangeness of these various thoughts and experiences, the patient spoke in an unemotional and detached fashion. His speech was somewhat disorganized and at times bordered on the incoherent. A diagnosis of a Schizophrenic Disorder in an active phase was made.

Residual Phase

Typically, patients shift gradually from an active phase of illness into a residual phase which is manifested by the same symptoms already described for the prodromal phase. But some remain chronically in an active phase, while others recover completely from an acute illness, with no residua. A patient who has had a definite schizophrenic disorder but recovers fully is considered, by convention, "in remission." If no recurrences then intervene over a period of 5 years without medication, the current diagnosis then is changed to No Mental Disorder. Some such patients, especially those still in remission, will suffer another attack, with the same varied set of subsequent outcomes. This is one aspect of the inherent heterogeneity of the schizophrenic syndrome already noted. Another is the existence of subtypes.

Subtypes

Several phenomenological subtypes of schizophrenic disorders are recognized. These have been designed to reflect the major cross-sectional syndromes, although it must be recognized that **these syndromes are not stable over time.**

The *disorganized subtype* is closely analogous to the older category of *hebephrenia*. Its clinical features are severe incoherence and the presence of flat, incongruous, or silly affect. Delusions and hallucinations tend to be fragmentary and poorly organized. This and the undifferentiated subtype tend to have the worst prognosis.

The *catatonic subtype* is characterized by marked involvement of the motor system in the direction of hyper- or hypoactivity. At times there is a relatively rapid alternation between excitement and stupor. Its short-term prognosis is good, but often it is succeeded by other subtypes.

The *paranoid subtype* is dominated by relative persistent persecutory or grandiose delusions, or those of jealousy, or hallucinations of similar content. Its onset tends to be later in life than in other subtypes. Although short-term treatment response tends to be undramatic, there is less tendency towards deterioration.

The *undifferentiated subtype* is characterized by prominent psychotic symptoms that cannot be classified in any of the previous subtypes, or includes the features of more than one.

The *residual subtype* is used to characterize those individuals who have an episode of unequivocal schizophrenic illness, whose current clinical picture no longer includes prominent psychotic symptoms. The most common manifestations take the form of emotional blunting, social withdrawal, eccentric behavior, and mild difficulties in communication. If delusions or hallucinations are present they have lost their affective intensity. This category is consistent with the concept of partial remission.

Differential Diagnosis

Two disorders particularly must be ruled out to make the diagnosis of a schizophrenic disorder: the organic and affective disorders. In addition, acute short-term illnesses are considered schizophreniform or reactive, as already noted (p. 55). Paranoid disorders will be considered in a later section of this chapter.

Organic Mental Disorders

These may present with symptoms such as delusions, hallucinations, incoherence, and affective changes which are suggestive of the schizophrenic disorders. This is particularly true for syndromes associated with amphetamine or phencyclidine (PCP). Sometimes it can be extremely difficult to differentiate the two disorders; and the proper differential diagnosis may require the passage of time. When confusion, disorientation, or memory impairment are present in the clinical picture, the diagnosis of Organic Mental Disorder must be considered. Acute brain syndromes can be life-threatening if not diagnosed and treated rapidly. Nevertheless, it is possible for an individual to have both simultaneously. Schizophrenics not infrequently abuse alcohol or drugs, and may suffer head injuries, etc.

Affective Disorders

This can be a difficult differentiation because most or even all the symptoms of a manic or depressive illness sometimes are present along with those of a schizophrenic disorder. The critical issue then is which symptoms developed first, and which are predominant. An affective disorder is only diagnosed when a depressive or manic (expansive, elevated, or irritable) mood preceded the schizophrenic symptoms and dominates the clinical picture. Unfortunately one may not be able to determine which symptoms occurred first.

Still more problematic, an acute manic episode and acute schizophrenia can look very much alike. Hyperactivity and excitement may occur in both. Manic flight of ideas, when severe, may appear as disorganized and incoherent speech. The irritability and anger of paranoid schizophrenia may be quite similar to that seen in a manic episode.

A history of good premorbid adjustment, a previous well-documented episode of affective disorder with complete recovery, or a family history of affective disorder are more likely in affective illness than schizophrenia. Clinically, the manic patient is more personally engaging. Manic exuberance and euphoria can be "infectious" and transiently entertaining. To an unfamiliar observer, the manic can seem almost normal and amusing, if overdoing it: like an immature version of one's self in an unusually "high" mood. In contrast, the sense of rapport with the schizophrenic is much more tenuous, and establishing a relationship difficult. The patient is often distant and not engaging, and seems not merely excited but "different." Finally, at times the only way to distinguish the two is with a trial of lithium treatment, which generally has no effect on the psychotic symptoms of schizophrenia, though it may modify the mood state.

Schizoaffective Disorder

This diagnosis is used in those few instances when there is a mixed picture wherein there is a full affective syndrome, but a preoccupation with those types of delusions or hallucinations characteristic of schizophrenia dominates the clinical picture; or where the absence of history makes it impossible to determine if dominant affective symptoms occurred before or after those of schizophrenia. This fudged diagnostic category is used for two reasons. A number of these patients seem to require treatment with both antipsychotic medication and an antidepressant or lithium. Also, grouping them separately will allow subsequent research directed to clarifying the fundamental nature of this disorder.

Atypical Psychosis

This diagnosis is reserved for those rare occasions in which some of the characteristic psychotic symptoms of a schizophrenic disorder are present, but no significant impairment in routine daily functioning exists. It remains unclear if this disorder is a milder form of the schizophrenic syndrome. Its management, however, is much the same.

Treatment

General Principles

The very heterogeneity of the schizophrenic disorders means that there must be a corresponding variety of treatments and that there can be no single or even preferred treatment. Furthermore, any single patient will show variability over time; and the treatment which is helpful at one point in the course of an illness may not be useful at another. It is essential, therefore, for the physician to remain flexible and to avoid dogmatism in the management of these patients. Furthermore, it is necessary to specify the goals of treatment clearly. Some clinicians, for example, seek the suppression of psychotic symptoms as a goal, while others desire to help the patient develop a reorganization of personality so as to make him presumably less vulnerable to further attacks. The choice of appropriate goals will vary also as a function of the phase and nature of a patient's illness, and especially its chronicity and the extent of functional deterioration which has already occurred. In the absence of specified therapeutic goals, it is impossible to assess the efficacy of any single treatment. Finally, there is no isomorphism between etiology and intervention. Somatic symptoms may respond to psychosocial interventions just as socially derived symptoms can respond to pharmacologic interventions.

In general, **the treatment of the schizophrenic patient should be undertaken by a psychiatrist** unless one is not available. The skills and time required for appropriate care are not likely to be readily available to the nonpsychiatrist. Clinical psychologists and other professionals trained in various forms of psychotherapy sometimes can be utilized, but there is an enormous advantage in having one person assume the complete responsibility for the patient's care. It is difficult enough for the normal person to relate to a team, and even more confusing for someone who is psychotic.

The **treatment of the acute phase almost always requires hospitalization.** This is helpful for the protection of the patient (and sometimes others); the maintenance of a less frightening, more stable environment; and better control of treatment. This permits more vigorous, rapid control of psychotic symptoms and thus diminishes the extent and duration of the disruption of the patient's life. It is not unusual for patients to do more harm to their social, interpersonal, and vocational lives by remaining in their environment than is produced by psychiatric hospitalization. Ordinarily, the main emphasis of treatment in the active phase is the elimination of psychotic symptoms, particularly those which drastically impair adaptation. Usually this requires antipsychotic medication.

In the residual phase, a probably prodromal phase, or when an acute illness is unusually mild, it is ordinarily possible to treat the patient in an ambulatory setting. The importance of social interventions increases dramatically at this time. The quality of the patient's social relatedness becomes far more critical when the supports of the hospital are withdrawn.

It is convenient to divide the available treatments into somatic and psychosocial approaches. The somatic approaches include pharmacologic agents, electroconvulsive therapy, insulin coma treatment, and surgical interventions. **The vast majority of patients will at one or another point in their treatment require pharmacologic intervention.** Several principles of drug treatment will be presented, but the details of pharmacologic management are to be found in Chapter 21.

Antipsychotic Medication

A large number of antipsychotic agents are available, and it is pointless to attempt to develop experience in the use of all of them. The clinician should learn how to use several drugs, and learn them well. While there is no evidence that any of the psychotic agents are inherently superior, idiosyncratic responses or failure to respond may necessitate the discontinuation of one drug and a trial with a different agent. Ideally, at least one drug from each of the major groups should be within the physician's armamentarium: The groups include the aliphatic, piperidine, and piperazine phenothiazines, as well as other antipsychotic compounds.

Before starting any of these, a comprehensive **medication history** must be obtained. This should include sensitivity, and the response and side effects of previous drugs. Where there is a family history of mental illness, inquiry should be made as to the responsiveness and sensitivity of those family members. Target symptoms and goals should be identified so that the dosage can be titrated against those specific clinical responses. Initial workup should also include baseline blood pressures (standing and reclining) and appropriate laboratory work including a complete blood count and liver profile, and an electrocardiogram in older patients.

Only one antipsychotic agent should be used at a time. There are very few clinical situations in which the simultaneous use of two or more is indicated. It is better practice to use adequate doses of one drug than suboptimal doses of more. Low dosages expose the patient to the risk of side effects without the potential benefit of improvement. The concomitant use of antidepressant or anxiolytic drugs is generally to be avoided. Few circumstances justify these combinations.

In hospitalized patients, it is wise to reach therapeutic doses reasonably rapidly over a period of 3 to 7 days. (There are exceptions, particularly when there are problems with the patient's general medical condition.) After control of the initial symptomatology, antipsychotic drugs are best administered once or twice a day. If the patient can tolerate the full dose at bedtime, this may be optimal because it is easy to remember and may help sleep. Furthermore, some immediate side effects are less likely to be troublesome if the patient is asleep. However, some patients require a split dose; and those who respond paradoxically and become aroused will do better to take all or most of the drug in the morning.

In hospitalized patients, it is often useful to use parenteral or liquid forms of medication because of problems in compliance. Even in the hospital, at least 20% of psychiatric patients discard usual oral medication without consuming it. The best way to enhance compliance is to develop a good doctor–patient relationship. In the absence of a therapeutic alliance, it is unrealistic to expect patients to cooperate in taking their medication. Blood or urine measures can be helpful in identifying patients who are not actually taking their medication. It is important to remember that parenteral medications are two to four times more powerful than the oral forms, and the dose must be corrected accordingly. Slower acting fluphenazine (both in the enanthate and decanoate forms) is not useful for the rapid control of psychotic symptoms. Its use is restricted primarily to the chronic management of patients who have difficulty in taking oral medication regularly.

It is usually necessary to treat a first schizophrenic episode or an acute exacerbation for 6 to 8 weeks with a particular drug before abandoning it as not helpful. In patients with more chronic illnesses lasting in excess of 2 years it may be necessary to give a particular drug as much as a 4- to 6-month trial.

There are occasions where "megadoses" are warranted: daily doses equivalent to 2 to 3 g of chlorpromazine. These are used in refractory patients under the age of 40 who have spent less than 10 years in hospital. Such patients, in general, should be managed in a hospital.

Anticholinergic side effects are common. Most are minor. But hypotension, usually of the postural type, can be dangerous, especially for patients with cardiovascular disease. Anti-alpha-adrenergic side effects also pose a danger to these patients, so that severe cardiovascular disease is a significant contraindication to antipsychotic medication. Extreme caution is warranted in patients with serious liver disorders. The use of neuroleptics in early pregnancy is a risk whose precise magnitude is not known. Extrapyramidal side effects are common and cause considerable problems in compliance. These are treated with anticholinergic antiparkinsonian drugs (e.g., benztropine mesylate 0.5 to 8 mg per day). Most psychopharmacologists oppose the use of these drugs in the absence of actual extrapyramidal symptoms. Their use increases overall anticholinergic effects and the dangers of these, including the possibility of delirium. If they are required, a trial of discontinuation is indicated after 2 to 3 months; almost 90% of such patients will then no longer require them.

The most serious side effect of neuroleptic medication is persistent *tardive dyskinesia*. This is particularly common in elderly patients. There is no established treatment. The key issue is prevention via use of the **lowest effective doses** of these drugs for only so long as they are required. Other side effects are described in Chapter 21.

Other Somatic Therapies

Electroconvulsive therapy (ECT) is rarely used any longer for schizophrenic disorders. Occasional patients who are resistant to medication and may require ECT; but for the vast majority neuroleptics are at least as effective, at a lower social cost.

Insulin coma treatment has almost dropped out of the therapeutic armamentarium; and the indications for psychosurgical intervention in the schizophrenic disorders are extraordinarily rare. For all practical purposes both can be ignored as treatment methods.

Psychosocial Approaches

Among the psychosocial approaches, **individual psychotherapy** remains extremely useful in selected cases. It is an opportunity for patients to enter into an intense, enduring, and stable human relationship. This intense social experience may be beneficial to the patient, and some of the benefits may be generalized to other social settings. Despite the relative paucity of convincing studies documenting its utility for schizophrenic disorders, there has been renewed interest in this technique in recent years.

Similarly, the use of **family therapy** has also received considerable attention, particularly in reducing the family's unrealistic expectations concerning the patient. Frequently, there are intrafamilial modes of interacting which can be harmful to the patient's adaptation. Family therapy can be useful in altering these. It is crucial to remember that family therapy is not a technique to find a scapegoat on whom to blame the patient's illness.

Group therapy can also be an effective way of mobilizing patients through peer support and pressure. A group also is an excellent opportunity to learn interpersonal and social skills which may be inadequately developed in a schizophrenic patient.

Many schizophrenic patients show serious social and vocational deficits during the residual phase of their illness. These deficits may go on for much of the patient's life unless there is active intervention to change the pattern. The neuroleptic agents have not been particularly helpful in changing the level of social adjustment or vocational competence. It is hardly surprising that we do not have drugs for influencing these learned skills. The need for **social and vocational rehabilitation** is both clear and compelling. In the absence of such interventions many people will be doomed to live marginal lives without full participation in the benefits of society. Even with them, fully 25% of the patients will be severely disabled psychosocially. We have been successful in shortening the duration of the illness but not as yet successful in reducing its human costs.

Paranoid Disorders[1]

These relatively uncommon disorders are traditionally considered as related to the schizophrenic disorders. However, the correctness of this assumption, or the nature of the relationship remain to be established. Certainly, there is a strong similarity to the paranoid subtype of schizophrenia.

The hallmark of these disorders is the presence of **persistent persecutory delusions or delusional jealousy.** These differ from schizophrenic delusions of similar content in being better organized and systematized. Moreover, other types of delusions, hallucinations which are more than fleeting, disorganization of thought, bizarre behavior, and impairment of general functioning are absent. Emotion and behavior may be disturbed in a fashion specifically consistent with the delusional beliefs. But other abnormal mood states are absent, as is a blunting or flattening of affect.

PARANOIA

The usual form of the disorder is insidious in onset, and chronic. The diagnosis is ordinarily not made unless the delusional system has been present in relatively stable form for at least 6 months.

---

[1]Dr. Donald Oken collaborated in writing this section.

ACUTE PARANOID DISORDERS

This acute state of less than 6 months duration, may be associated with somewhat greater instability of the delusional beliefs and more sudden episodes of emotional or behavioral outbursts arising from these. This may be difficult initially to distinguish from a schizophreniform disorder or an early phase of a schizophrenic disorder; and if volatile emotional behavior does not soon decrease or the delusions do not become stabilized, one of these diagnosis is probably the correct one.

SHARED PARANOID DISORDER

This fascinating rare condition arises in an emotionally unstable person who is in close, enduring contact with another person(s) who has an established mental disorder with persecutory delusions. The condition disappears with psychotherapeutic support and insight once separation from the "contagious" other(s) is effected, but may be persistent as long as the direct relationship continues.

Differential Diagnosis

In addition to the **Schizophrenic Disorders,** persecutory and jealous delusions are quite common also in the **Organic Mental Disorders.** These disorders are differentiated in the same fashion as they are from schizophrenia by the concomitant presence of disturbances in the cognitive sphere and/or levels of consciousness. (These findings are discussed in Chapter 4.) Grandiose, expansive delusions are not a feature of paranoid disorders, but suggest the presence of a *manic* episode or a schizophrenic disorder. In a *paranoid personality disorder,* suspiciousness, jealousy, and feelings of persecution are less intense and not delusional.

Course and Treatment

Paranoia is a chronic illness. Although deterioration is usually minimal, the delusional state is typically persistent and impervious to treatment. Antipsychotics can be tried but rarely help, and usually are refused. Psychotherapy is directed to helping the patient gain control over his behavior so that he does not act on his delusions; and some amelioration of their intensity sometimes can be achieved. Except in certain highly specialized forms of psychotherapy (to be performed only by experts) delusions are not confronted or challenged or argued with; rather one tries to work around these to discuss behavior or other aspects of the patient's life.

Acute paranoid disorders are significantly more responsive to antipsychotic medication and psychotherapy, especially early in their course.

The longer their duration, the poorer the prognosis. Most of these patients stabilize into a chronic paranoia.

Although **danger to others** is less frequent than commonly believed, it is a realistic issue which the doctor must constantly keep in mind. Hospitalization may be required to protect others. Care must be taken by staff to protect themselves from sudden outbursts of rage over confinement or directed at staff members who are added to the delusional system. Patients with Acute Paranoid Disorders are especially unpredictable. But even seemingly stable chronic patients may suddenly become violent. Driven by their delusional beliefs, these patients can be extraordinarily clever in making plans to effect escape or retribution. A special problem arises in the patient whose delusions are well-circumscribed and kept hidden from others, so that they are able to convince legal authorities that there is no basis for involuntary hospitalization. If the psychiatrist determines that these patients do constitute a danger to identifiable others, he may need to report this fact to the authorities and/or potential victim. In this rare situation, the physician should consult his attorney about specific obligations and the freedom to abrogate confidentiality in that jurisdiction.

Additional Readings

Bleuler E: Dementia Praecox or the Group of the Schizophrenias. New York, International Universities Press, 1950

Cancro R: Overview of schizophrenia, in Comprehensive Textbook of Psychiatry—III. Edited by Kaplan HI, Freedman AM, Sadcock BJ. Baltimore, Williams & Wilkins, 1980, Chapter 15, pp 1093–1104

Diagnostic and Statistical Manual, 3rd ed. (DSM III). Washington, DC, American Psychiatric Association, 1980

Lehmann H: Schizophrenia: Clinical features, in Comprehensive Textbook of Psychiatry—III. Edited by Kaplan HI, Freedman AM, Sadock BJ. Baltimore, Williams & Wilkins, 1980, Chapter 15, pp 1153–1192

Oppenheimer H: Clinical Psychiatry. New York, Harper & Row, 1971, pp 206–271

Weiner H: Schizophrenia: Etiology, in Comprehensive Textbook of Psychiatry—III. Edited by Kaplan HL, Freedman AM, Sadcock BJ. Baltimore, Williams & Wilkins, 1980, Chapter 15, pp 1121–1152

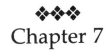

Chapter 7

Affective Disorders
Depressions and Mania

Gerald L. Klerman

The purpose of this chapter is to provide descriptions of the affective disorders, their causes and development, with particular attention to differential diagnosis of the range of patients likely to be seen in medical settings. This information makes it possible to identify a sequence of decisions involved in the doctor–patient interaction from the first contact, where assessment should lead to diagnosis, through the treatment of acute episodes into issues of long-term treatment. To a considerable extent, the complexity of the decisions required is a tribute to recent progress in the understanding and treatment of these disorders. Better understanding of psychopathology makes history taking and diagnosis more difficult and the availability of many effective treatments, both biological and psychological, similarly presents the clinician with a broad range of choices.

Diagnosis of Affective Disorders

The new (1980) *Diagnostic and Statistical Manual of Mental Disorders* (DSM-III) defines affective disorders as a group whose **essential feature is a disturbance of mood, accompanied by a full or partial manic or depressive syndrome, that is not due to any other physical or mental disorder.** The term *mood* refers to a prolonged emotion that colors the whole psychic life; it generally involves either depression or elation. The manic and depressive syndromes consist of characteristic symptoms that tend to occur together, including disturbances of mood.

Clinical diagnosis of manic and depressive episodes are made both easier and more difficult by virtue of the fact that **the clinical mood states represent more intense manifestations of aspects of normal emotional life.** All human beings sometimes experience pleasure and happiness, and periods of sadness, disappointment and discouragement. This contributes to the physician's better empathic understanding of the experience of both the manic and depressive patient. At the same time, it can make diagnosis and clinical management more difficult because the apparent normality of the emotional states may lead the clinician to underestimate the severity of the dysfunction; and often there is difficulty in demarcating the normal range from the clinical state.

The current trend, embodied in DSM-III, is to diagnose the manic and depressive syndromes on the basis of manifest descriptive psychopathology, i.e., those symptoms and behaviors that the patient presents during the current episode and particularly at the time of clinical interview. This descriptive characterization is made independent of presumed etiology, whether biological, developmental, or psychodynamic.

Having made the diagnosis of either a manic or depressive syndrome, a series of questions then arise as to further classifying the particular disorder. There is no one affective disorder. Rather **there are a series of manic and depressive syndromes** which have different etiologic and pathogenic components, and which merit different treatment responses. While there is no universal agreement as to the best manner for subclassifying these, significant recent progress has led to both theoretically sound classificatory systems and guidelines for decisions regarding treatment and management.

A suggested schema for classifying affective disorders is shown in Fig. 1. **The major distinction is between primary and secondary affective disorders.** This distinction is based on the chronology and presence of associated illnesses (Robins and Guze, 1972). Primary affective disorders are those occurring in patients who have been well, or whose only previous psychiatric illnesses were mania or depression. Secondary affective disorders occur in mentally ill patients who have another psychiatric or physical illness. This approach attempts to separate out affective disorders that occur in the presence of other disorders, defining the residual category as primary disorders. Although the primary–secondary distinction is conceptually clear-cut, a number of practical problems arise in differentiating mania or depression that occur in association either with other clinical psychiatric disorders such as schizophrenia, anxiety, or alcoholism, or with systemic medical diseases such as endocrine disturbances, tumors, or viral infections. Drug-induced depression or mania caused by antihypertensive drugs, corticosteroids, or other agents constitute another large group of secondary disorders.

The clinical importance of the primary–secondary distinction becomes most evident in medical settings such as general hospitals where there

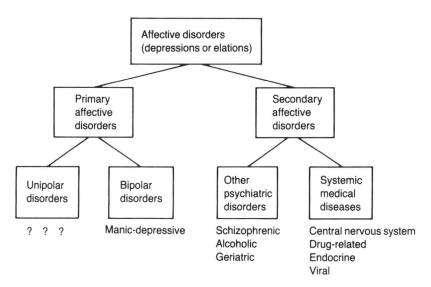

Figure 1. Suggested nosology of affective disorders.

are a substantial number of patients with medical disorders. A significant percentage of these will manifest a depressive syndrome. The importance of this is twofold. First, **careful differential diagnosis is essential,** so as not to miss a possible hormonal condition or viral infection such as viral hepatitis or mononucleosis. Second, where the depression is secondary to drugs such as antihypertensives (e.g., rauwolfia derivatives, or Aldomet), it can often be relieved by discontinuation or lowered dosage of the medication. Treatment of these secondary depressions requires close collaboration between a psychiatrist and the medical specialist, and knowledge of the interactions between drugs used in the treatment of medical illnesses and those used for psychiatric disturbances.

A second major subclassification divides the unipolar form of affective disorder from the bipolar form. The latter is distinguished by the prior occurrence of a manic episode, regardless of whether the current episode is depression or mania. There is considerable evidence of genetic, familial, personality, biochemical, physiological, and pharmacological differences between bipolar and unipolar disorders. Patients with bipolar disorder have a far higher frequency of positive family history than did patients with only depression. They also usually respond well to lithium, and are more likely to develop hypomanic responses to tricyclic antidepressants than patients with nonbipolar depression. The latter, on the other hand, have the most favorable responses to the tricyclics.

Classification of the type of disorder should be only one phase of

assessment, which is the total process of collecting information relevant to diagnosis and treatment. These data should include a comprehensive psychiatric, medical, personal, and social history, as well as a complete physical examination with relevant laboratory studies. Among the most important considerations prior to initiating treatment is the assessment of the patient's family and social resources and environmental supports. In practice, most treatment decisions are determined not only by the nature of the patient's psychopathology or severity of illness, but also by the extent and availability of social support systems, especially the family.

The Depressions

Depressions are the most common psychiatric condition that clinicians are likely to encounter in adult patients. Approximately 15 to 30% of all adults experience an episode of depressive disorder at some time during their lives. Depressions occur about twice as frequently among women as men, and often occur during the highly productive years of young adulthood.

Depressive Syndrome

Between 10 and 35% of all patients seen in office visits or admitted to a hospital will have either depressive symptoms accompanying their medical or surgical illnesses. In perhaps 10 to 25%, the depression will be the primary condition. Differential diagnosis may be difficult because **the patient may not emphasize emotional symptoms but rather uses various bodily complaints** (such as sleep difficulty, backache, headache, or change in menstruation) as the "ticket of admission" to the medical care system. Careful attention to the existence of these so-called masked depressions or "bodily equivalents" will improve the quality of care and reduce the excess utilization of expensive X-ray and laboratory tests. Thorough but gentle probing about the patient's emotional life, interpersonal relations, sleep difficulty, and changes in lifestyle will facilitate unmasking the depressive mood, and clarify the diagnostic problem.

The first important decision is whether or not the patient meets the criteria for the depressive syndrome. **The predominant symptom of the depressive syndrome is a feeling of sadness.** Concomitant with this inner distress, the patient may report one or more of the following: **cognitive manifestations,** such as thoughts of worthlessness, guilt, helplessness, and hopelessness; **physiological disturbances** in sleep, appetite, sexual interest, and autonomic nervous system or gastrointestinal functioning; **behavioral changes** manifested by reduced desire and ability to perform usual social roles; and **possibly suicidal ideation,** confusion, hallucinations, and delusions. Usually several of these symptoms occur together to form the syndrome.

There is no clear boundary between normal mood and clinical depression meriting intervention. Feelings of sadness, disappointment, and frustration are a component of the human condition. However, when the sadness interferes with normal functioning, medical intervention may be helpful. In general, depression is recognized as pathological by virtue of its intensity, pervasiveness, persistence, and interference with usual social and physiological functioning.

Diagnostically, patients with depressions present problems at two other boundaries: anxiety on one side and schizophrenia on the other. Many forms of depression occur in patients who also experience symptoms of anxiety, tension, insomnia, and restlessness. Clinicians frequently must distinguish patients who suffer predominantly from anxiety states with associated depressed mood from those who suffer from a predominantly depressive reaction in which anxiety is a frequent concomitant. It is also important to distinguish between those with schizophrenic disorders, especially schizoaffective states (both of which include disturbances in thought processes) so that appropriate pharmacologic intervention can be prescribed. In the elderly especially, the distinction from organic brain syndromes and somatic conditions may be difficult (see Chapter 12).

Specific Treatments for Depression

The majority of depressive patients can be treated on ambulatory basis with the use of drugs or psychotherapy, or both. The doctor should be familiar with the range of treatments available, and skilled in the use of the standard drugs, alone or combined with specific forms of psychotherapy. Just as important as specific therapeutic techniques is the development of a general psychotherapeutic approach toward the patient—a process emphasizing support, empathy, and a positive attitude, while offering substantive amelioration and longer-term growth possibilities rather than simple reassurances.

ANTIDEPRESSANT DRUG TREATMENTS

The pharmacologic treatment of depression has undergone major changes since the introduction of the phenothiazines and the tricyclic antidepressants in the late 1950s. Since this topic is covered in more detail in Chapter 21, only brief summary statements will be made here.

This treatment involves a selection among a range of compounds with varying efficacy, falling into two major classes: the tricyclic antidepressants and the MAO inhibitors. In addition, large numbers of patients in clinical practice receive antianxiety drugs, particularly diazepam and other chlordiazepoxides. In recent years less attention has been given to the use of the phenothiazines because of the appropriate concern about tardive dyskinesia as an adverse consequence.

In patients with manifest **delusional forms** of psychotic depression, the evidence indicates that tricyclics alone will not produce a treatment response. Either treatment combining a tricyclic with a phenothiazine, or ECT is called for.

Similar **caution is required in the use of tricyclics for patients with a history of mania or hypomania** (bipolar illness). Both the MAO inhibitors and the tricyclics are prone to overstimulate the CNS of such patients, and push them over into a manic or excited state. In fact, in one large study, bipolar patients treated only with a tricyclic had a poorer outcome than the placebo group because of the number who developed a manic state as an adverse effect. Caution is required in using a tricyclic; if the history of bipolar illness is clear-cut, the combination of lithium and a tricyclic may be desirable.

In the use of tricyclics alone, the main guide to selection of patients is the presence of "endogenous" symptom features during the acute episode. In DSM III, this symptom picture is termed *melancholia*. Symptoms such as early morning awakening, and other sleep difficulty, diurnal variation, weight loss, guilt, agitation, and retardation are predictors of good response to tricyclics. On the other hand, the presence or absence of a recent life event or preexisting neurotic personality difficulties does not bear any predictive relationship to the response to tricyclics. Clinical folklore still recommends that tricyclics not be used for neurotic depressions or for patients with long-standing characterological or personality difficulties. Recent research indicates that this is an inaccurate guide. The important consideration should not be the presence or absence of a life event as a precipitant, social stress, or preexisting personality and characterological difficulties, but rather the nature of the presenting symptoms, particularly those characterized as endogenous (termed *melancholia* in DSM III).

There is less certainty for those patients whose depression does not fit the endogenous picture. Sometimes these are called atypical or hysterical depressions. There is some suggestion that these patients respond well to MAO inhibitors, but further research is called for.

THE PSYCHOTHERAPIES

It is important to distinguish between general psychological management and specific psychotherapeutic methods.

Psychotherapeutic Management. The development of rapport, empathy, and understanding is basic to all doctor–patient transactions. Special problems arise, however, in relating optimally to depressed patients.

During the acute episode, the doctor should be active, available, and flexible in his approach. Nondirective psychotherapy is contraindicated, since patients may interpret this approach as rejection. **During diagnostic interviews, the doctor should actively elicit information, particularly that concerning possible suicidal trends, thoughts, and impulses.** Other vital information include sleep changes, appetite and weight changes, bodily functions, sexual fantasies and performance, and various fears. This information can and should be sought in a friendly but persistent manner—an interview rather than an interrogation. The doctor should be flexible with regard to his appointment schedule. Patients need not always be seen for long periods (e.g., 50 minutes). It may be useful to see the patient more than once each week for brief periods. If the patient has episodes of anxiety and panic, he should be made comfortable about telephoning the doctor to obtain temporary support. One should not hesitate to see the relatives, both to elicit background information and, particularly in suicidal patients, to obtain their understanding, cooperation and assistance.

Particular problems arise for patients who ask for reassurance. ("Tell me I'm not losing my mind"; "Tell me I'm going to get better.") **It is not always therapeutically useful to reassure the patient automatically.** Members of the family have been attempting this for weeks. Rather, the patient should be asked, "What do you mean by losing your mind?" The response may be, "I feel like jumping out the window," or, "I may want to divorce my husband." Before providing simple reassurance, the doctor must probe the underlying fears and anxieties; the source may not be self-evident or even conscious.

Another management problem concerns **the response to complaints of bodily dysfunction.** Depressed patients frequently complain of difficulty in sleeping, appetite loss, fatigue, headache, backache, cramps, constipation, and other problems. Too often these patients are told by physicians, "It's all in your mind." This does themselves and their patients disservice. The research evidence is to the contrary; depression is a psychosomatic state. Dysfunctions of the neuroendocrine and autonomic nervous systems in fact exist in depression; and patients perceive alterations in their bodily functions that are reversible as the depression is alleviated. The doctor who inquires carefully about bodily dysfunctions and attempts to explain the nature of psychosomatic relationships will often strengthen his therapeutic alliance with the patient.

Specific Psychotherapeutic Techniques. A number of specific forms of psychotherapy are useful during the acute depressive episode. These include psychoanalysis, behavior modification, group therapy, family therapy, and psychodynamically oriented individual psychotherapy.

An extensive review of the literature describing the efficacy of psychotherapy alone and in interaction with drug therapy for treating depression was done by Weissman (1979). This study revealed that the effects of psychotherapy were strongest in areas related to problems in living, social functioning, and interpersonal relationships.

Individual psychotherapy based on psychodynamic (psychoanalytic) principles remains the most widely used form of psychotherapy. Although systematic, controlled studies do not exist, clinical observations strongly support the value of this form of therapy during both acute and long-term treatments. Indirect support for its efficacy can be found in the literature on other forms of psychotherapy. In actual practice, most individual psychotherapy conducted one or more times a week uses combinations of cognitive, behavioral, and interpersonal with psychodynamic exploratory techniques.

The usefulness of psychoanalysis in acute depressions remains controversial. No systematic or controlled studies of the outcome of psychoanalysis in the treatment of depression exist. On the basis of clinical observations, psychoanalysis seems indicated for neurotic depressions in individuals with long-standing personality disorders. It is less clearly indicated as primary treatment for patients with bipolar manic depressive illness or those who have had severe recurrent depressions. Other specific psychotherapies include cognitive and behavioral, family and marital, and group psychotherapy.

Cognitive behavioral psychotherapy developed recently as a specific technique for dealing with patients with problems of self-esteem and misperception, who often blame themselves unduly and underestimate their ability to perform. Research has demonstrated that depressed patients suffer from low self-esteem and difficulties in interpersonal relations, particularly in the context of social situations, families, and small groups. Several new forms of individual, family, and group therapies have been derived from studies of cognitive, behavioral, and social learning aspects of the depressed patient's psychological functioning.

Group therapy that assists patients in their social roles and facilitates the development of social skills has proved useful, particularly where patients receive a mirror image or feedback of the impact of their interpersonal behavior on others. This often reverses the social skills deficit of depressed patients. Research indicates that many depressed patients are unable to obtain the social rewards that other people elicit in group situations.

Interpersonal psychotherapy is aimed at improving the patient's interpersonal relations. Whether conducted by psychiatrists or social workers, good evidence suggests that it can improve the patient's coping ability in interpersonal difficulties—particularly in marriage, family relations, and childrearing.

Marital issues and their treatment are a particular problem for women in today's culture. Epidemiologic research has shown a rapid increase of depressions in young women, particularly well-educated women. Their depression seems related to the conflictful position of women in contemporary society and their wish to redress what they feel to be inequities in the conventional marriage relationship. Current forms of marital therapy do not merely treat the depressed women; rather, group or couples methods are employed to improve the modes of communication and the transaction between patient and spouse.

It is important to distinguish between psychotherapeutic techniques useful in the management of the acute symptomatic episode from those most helpful in long-term treatment. During the symptomatic acute stage, the emphasis is on symptom relief to facilitate the patient's return to premorbid social and occupational adjustment. It is doubtful whether methods such as psychoanalysis or other uncovering techniques are effective here. On the other hand, as the acute symptomatic state subsides, exploration of current interpersonal relations, intrapsychic conflicts, and antecedent developmental experiences is indicated. This form of long-term therapy seems most appropriate for patients with problems of self-esteem, interpersonal difficulties, and conflicts involving guilt, hostility, and sexuality.

Combined Chemotherapy and Psychotherapy. In practice, large numbers of patients are treated with drugs in combination with psychotherapy. Numerous controlled studies indicate that **the combination is almost always more effective than either component alone,** particularly with more severely ill patients, such as manic-depressive and severely impaired neurotic patients. The rationale is that each appears to act on different targets. Psychotherapy is most beneficial in enhancing social effectiveness and personality functioning, whereas drugs are most effective in influencing the pathophysiology of symptom formation, such as sleep disturbance, loss of energy, and loss of sexual drive.

There are three groups of patients for whom this combined regimen is specifically indicated. The first includes patients who have been on maintenance treatment with lithium or tricyclics. As mood symptoms subside, problems of irritability appear; and issues previously ignored, such as childrearing and marriage, become a focus of family attention. These problems are well addressed by psychotherapeutic intervention. Patients with neurotic character problems and other long-standing personality maladjustments form the second group. These patients do not seem to do well on drugs alone, and may benefit from added psychotherapy by exploring the developmental antecedents of the problems, while simultaneously receiving support and alleviation of mood and somatic symptoms. Finally, combined therapy is useful for patients with depressions that arise in the context of marital conflicts.

ELECTROCONVULSIVE THERAPY (ECT)

Electroconvulsive therapy (variously called "shock" or "convulsive" therapy) was first developed from experience with metrazol-induced convulsions. The induction of convulsions, whether by chemical or electrical means, is associated with relief of acute depression. The CNS mechanism for this action is unknown. It does not seem to require peripheral muscular contractions, since the therapeutic action will continue even if these are blocked (by the use of a muscle relaxant such as Anectine). There does appear to be some specificity in the location, since other placements will not produce as good a clinical response as when the electrode is over the temporal–parietal area, activating the motor cortex. A number of hypotheses have been proposed; but the main basis for the use of ECT remains empirical. Numerous carefully controlled trials have demonstrated the superiority of ECT over no treatment, and as effective—if not slightly superior—to the tricyclics.

For severely depressed patients, especially those with marked psychomotor retardation or agitation, suicidal drive or delusions, ECT is the treatment of first choice. It is also useful for patients who do not respond to other treatments. ECT is of great value for patients with intense suicidal drive, for whom one does not wish to wait 5 to 15 days for drug treatment to take effect, for the severely depressed, and for those patients whose medical condition contraindicated the use of drugs.

The most frequent adverse effect of ECT is memory loss. While usually temporary and rarely severe, this is distressing to the patient. But unilateral electrode placements have minimized this effect. And other refinements in technology, and limitations on the frequency and number of treatments have increased the efficacy of ECT, while substantially ameliorating its side effects.

The decision to use ECT always should be based upon the evaluation of a carefully trained and experienced psychiatrist. Usually there are one or more psychiatrists available with sufficient experience in both the diagnostic considerations as well as the actual administration of this procedure. The administration of ECT should be limited to the hospital setting; and ideally requires a team including an anesthesiologist or anesthetist.

Clinical Management of the Acute Depressive Episode

In the practical management of acute depression, assessment of severity is often useful. **In mild depression,** either no drug treatment or the administration of tricyclics with or without psychotherapy are viable options. Psychotherapy alone is most used with these patients. **Moderately depressed patients** are often helped by antidepressant drugs used conjointly with psychotherapy. **The clearest indication for tricyclic drugs is in endogenous depressive illness.** The tricyclics are the class of drug with the greatest efficacy and relative margin of safety; however, an MAO inhibitor may be used. For patients with a history of manic episodes or persistent elation, lithium should be strongly considered in addition to tricyclics. Drug treatment should be continued for a period of at least several weeks after complete symptom relief, and then tapered off.

In current practice, most patients can be treated effectively on an outpatient basis. However, for severely or extremely depressed patients, hospitalization must be considered, especially if suicidal ideation, delusions, or serious medical complications are present. The **decision between hospitalization and outpatient treatment may depend on the assessment of the risk of suicide.** ECT is usually the most effective treatment of severe depression. Phenothiazines may also be helpful in patients who are experiencing hallucinations or delusions. Difficult, complex, or unresponsive cases of depression require consultation by experts in psychotherapy or psychopharmacology.

Long-term Treatment of Depression

The decision to begin **maintenance therapy** involves the number, type, and severity of affective episodes; social consequences of the illness; the patient's wishes, personality and reliability; medical issues; and family history. If the nature of the depression is severe and the social consequences of relapse great, long-term treatment should be considered. In general, the more frequent the number of previous episodes, whether treated or not (or hospitalized or not), and the briefer the interval between episodes, the more suitable the patient is for long-term treatment. If long-term treatment is necessary, treatment with either the tricyclic antidepressants or lithium, alone or in conjunction with some form of psychotherapy, is suggested.

Mania

Mania is much less common than depression; it is estimated that approximately 10% of manic depressives are bipolar. Only a small fraction of bipolar patients experience recurrent mania in the absence of discernible episodes of depression. The incidence of mania is about equal in the two sexes. The modal age of onset of bipolar disease is below 30. In contrast, depression occurs about twice as often in women, and the peak age of onset is later.

The Manic Syndrome

For the diagnosis of mania, most current classification schemes require the **presence of either elation or irritability plus a variable number of behavioral or somatic symptoms:** pressure of speech, flight of ideas, racing thoughts, grandiosity, distractibility, poor judgment, insomnia without fatigue, increased energy, weight loss, and motor and/or sexual hyperactivity.

Recent clinical experience indicates a spectrum of manias. Use of the term mania encompasses the spectrum of elated mood from normal states to extremes of delirious mania, as follows:

1. Normal states: happiness, pleasure, joy
2. Neurotic elations: cyclothymic personality, hypomanic personality
3. Hypomania (nonpsychotic)
4. Mania (psychotic); delusions or other manifestations of impaired reality testing
5. "Delirious mania": maniacal overactivity, hostile attitude toward others, destruction of property, assaultiveness toward others, paranoid delusions

There is little disagreement about the diagnosis of the core syndrome, but several boundary problems present difficulties. The principal one is with normality in the form of cyclothymic or hypomanic episodes. Often, mild manic episodes are experienced by the patient as pleasant, desirable and sexually productive, and will not be sufficiently disruptive to cause the patient to present for psychiatric treatment. But family members or co-workers may be disturbed by the patient's mood swings and behavior fluctuations, and recommend treatment. In diagnosing mania, it is important to ascertain whether or not the return to normal from a prior depressive episode is experienced as a relief from depression, or whether there are clear signs of euphoria, increased activity and poor judgment, in which case it should be adjudged a manic disorder.

Another major boundary problem exists between mania and schizophrenic states. Patients who are manic and who have grossly disorganized psychotic behavior often are judged to have typical symptoms of schizophrenic disorders as well. But there is considerable debate as to whether these states should be regarded as variants of mania, of schizophrenia, or as a separate diagnostic entity: schizoaffective disorders.

Treatment of the Acute Episode

Shaw (1979) has suggested a series of guidelines for the treatment of acute mania depending on the severity of the episode. For **patients with mild elation, including hypomania, the choice of treatment is lithium,** preferably administered on an outpatient basis. **In moderately severe mania, a combination of lithium and an oral neuroleptic may be necessary.** The neuroleptic can be withdrawn when a noticeable reduction in mania occurs. **In severely disturbed patients, administration of neuroleptics, perhaps by intramuscular route, may be the**

treatment of choice. Lithium by itself is not always an effective and practical treatment for the socially disruptive behavior.

Initial judgments about whether to provide treatment at home or in a hospital setting depend on the assessment of the severity of the manic reaction, the degree of interference with the individual's functioning at home, work, and other social situations, and the strength of family and social supports. The most difficult treatment problems for patients with acute manic episodes is to rapidly bring the overactive and socially dysfunctional behavior under control. In severe forms, this will usually require hospitalization, particularly if the patient is destructive of property, threatening to persons, or manifesting psychotic exaggeration, grandiosity or paranoid trends. It is possible sometimes to manage milder forms of hypomania and mania on an ambulatory basis; but this requires considerable experience, the availability of a cooperative patient and a patient, and firm family setting.

For rapid management of the behavioral disruptive features, the use of a neuroleptic drug, particularly one of the phenothiazines or haloperidol, has been shown to be highly effective. Neuroleptics are more useful in the acute early phase than lithium for two reasons. They bring the behavioral manifestations of excitement, overactivity, and grandiosity rapidly under control; and monitoring of their blood levels is not required.

LITHIUM

The efficacy of lithium in the treatment of acute mania is well established; and it is the treatment of first choice. Its chief advantage is that it normalizes the patient.

Before lithium is started, laboratory tests of renal and thyroid function should be done to provide baseline values for the assessment of drug side effects. Starting dose is approximately 1800 mg/day, but should be lower in elderly patients. Dosage should be gradually increased. **However, monitoring by frequent blood level measures is essential.** Therapeutic blood levels are between 0.6 and 1.2 mEq/liter but can vary widely. Blood levels should be maintained below 1.6 mEq/liter unless treatment is conducted by an expert. A disadvantage of lithium is the delay involved in achieving adequate blood levels and, hence, therapeutic effect. Improvement typically occurs within 8 to 10 days.

The most common side effects are gastrointestinal irritation, a fine hand tremor, fatigue, drowsiness, and sometimes polyuria. More severe toxic reactions are nausea, diarrhea, vomiting, augmented tremor, cogwheel rigidity, aphasia, delirium, seizures, thyroid toxicity, polyuria, polydipsia, and possible renal damage. Lithium toxicity can be managed by discontinuing the use of the drug and increasing fluid intake. Lithium is not recommended during pregnancy or for patients with severe renal or cardiovascular disease.

NEUROLEPTICS

Both chlorpromazine and haloperidol have been compared to lithium for the treatment of acute mania. Studies show that these neuroleptics control the hyperactivity and excitement of the acutely manic patient more rapidly than does lithium. In practice, neuroleptics are most useful for highly active, psychotic and disturbed patients where rapid control of disruptive behavior is required. Then they can be cautiously tapered off.

Long-term Treatment of Mania

Lithium is the agent of choice for long-term treatment because of its prophylactic effects. It has been shown convincingly to reduce recurrences of both manic and depressive episodes in bipolar patients and to modify the quality of those subsequent episodes which do occur. The question of when to use lithium on a long-term basis depends on the severity of the affective disorder, the frequency of episodes, the patient's wishes, and his reliability for taking medication regularly.

Manic patients are traditionally difficult candidates for psychotherapy; however, recent reports indicate that psychotherapy and counseling (in conjunction with lithium maintenance treatment) may be useful in enhancing lithium compliance and improving long-term outcome.

The secondary effects of mania can be particularly disruptive to family functioning and result in high levels of marital discord. Couples group therapy can be helpful in these situations. Since bipolar illness has a strong genetic component, genetic counseling may also be an important contribution to helping patients cope with affective disorders and plan for the future.

Conclusions

Affective disorders, especially depression, are the most common psychiatric disorders that clinicians are likely to encounter. A number of efficacious treatments are available. In many patients, drug treatments and psychotherapy, alone or in combination, produce a rapid rate of improvement, ameliorate many of the pathological symptoms, and facilitate resumption of normal everyday activities. Given the availability of those various types of treatment provides the clinician with both the challenge and the opportunity to **tailor treatment decisions to the individual patient** and to combine humanistic skills with flexibility and pragmatism.

Additional Readings

Beck AT: Depression: Clinical, Experimental and Theoretical Aspects. New York, Harper & Row, 1969

Diagnostic and Statistical Manual of Mental Disorders, 3rd ed. (DSM III). Washington, DC, American Psychiatric Association, 1980

Klerman GL: Overview of affective disorders, in Comprehensive Textbook of Psychiatry, 3rd ed. Edited by Kaplan HI, Freedman AM, Sadock BJ. Baltimore, Williams & Wilkins, 1980, Chapter 19.1, pp 1305–1319

Mandel MM, Klerman GL: Clinical use of antidepressants, stimulants, tricyclics and monoamine oxidase inhibitors, in Principles of Psychopharmacology, 2nd ed. Edited by Clark W. New York, Academic, 1978, pp 537–551

Paykel ES, Coppen A: Psychopharmacology of Affective Disorders. New York, Oxford University Press, 1979

Robins E, Guze S: Classification of affective disorders: The primary-secondary, the endogenous-reactive, and the neurotic-psychotic concepts, in Recent Advances in the Psychobiology of the Depressive Illness. Edited by Williams TA, Katz MM, Shield JA. Washington, DC, Department of Health, Education, and Welfare, 1972, pp 283–293

Chapter 8

Neuroses and Personality Disorders

John C. Nemiah

Neuroses and personality disorders, along with the psychoses, constitute the three major classes of psychiatric syndromes. Neuroses may be found in conjunction with behavior patterns that characterize the personality disorders, but are further distinguished by symptoms specific to the several diagnostic categories into which they are divided.

Neuroses

General Features of Neurosis

In contrast to psychoses, the neuroses produce a less severe and less extensive disruption of the mind's functions than that brought about by major psychiatric illness. Neurotic patients generally maintain their capacity for reality testing—that is, they are able to discern the difference between external reality and internal thoughts, feelings, and fantasies. Furthermore, except in certain hysterical states, there is no major distortion of perceptions in the form of hallucinations and illusions. Neurotic phenomena are generally experienced as being *ego-alien*—as undesirable symptoms foreign to the sense of self.

Etiology

Neurotic symptoms may be thought of in psychological terms as being the result of psychological conflict. Certain inner impulses (mainly sexual and aggressive in nature), as well as the feelings and fantasies related to them, are viewed as unacceptable by the ego, which imposes controls on their emergence into conscious experience and expression by erecting ego defenses in opposition to them. Repression, the major ego defense, renders the unacceptable mental contents unconscious. Though removed from the sphere of conscious experience, the now-unconscious impulses, feelings, and fantasies still press for discharge and may produce ego-alien symptoms that represent disguised compromises between the impulses and the forces of the controlling defenses.

A brief example from Pierre Janet may make this psychodynamic model of symptom formation more intelligible. A young woman suffered from hysterical blindness in the left eye and anesthesia of the left side of her face. Under hypnosis, she recalled a long-forgotten (i.e., repressed) memory of being forced as a little girl to sleep in the same bed with a companion, the left side of whose face was covered with impetiginous scabs. Although the sight of her friend's face revolted her, her pleas not to share the bed were ignored. Shortly thereafter, she too developed facial impetigo. When this subsequently healed, the hysterical blindness and anesthesia remained as sequelae. The memories of this painful event, vividly recollected under hypnosis, were totally beyond the patient's recall in her normal waking state. The effect, however, of the unconscious memories was evident in the physical hysterical symptoms which, though totally ego-alien and beyond voluntary recall, graphically represented and recreated the essence of the "forgotten" painful experience. Based on his understanding of the psychological origin and structure of her symptom, Janet performed specific psychotherapeutic maneuvers that changed the painful quality of the patient's unconscious memories and resulted in a dramatic, lasting disappearance of her hysterical symptoms.

In the description of the various forms of neurotic illness that follows, it will not be possible to elaborate the specific psychodynamic mechanisms of each. Suffice it to say that the basic model of psychological conflict outlined is applicable to all; and that individual differences between the neuroses result from the use of a variety of ego defenses auxiliary to the basic defense of repression, the form of each neurosis being determined by the nature of the defenses employed. It should further be emphasized that, in addition to psychological mechanisms, other factors (especially biological and genetic) are important in the production of neurotic symptoms, although our knowledge of these causal elements is less extensive and well defined.

Neurotic Syndromes

The class of neuroses comprises: (1) anxiety neurosis; (2) phobic neurosis; (3) obsessive–compulsive neurosis; (4) depressive neurosis; and (5) hysterical neurosis, (a) conversion type, and (b) dissociative type. These constitute the major neurotic syndromes. In addition, there are three neurotic disorders that are relatively uncommon: (1) neurasthenic neurosis; (2) depersonalization; (3) hypochondriasis.

It should be noted that the classificatory scheme followed here is that of the **second** edition (1968) of the *Diagnostic and Statistical Manual of Mental Disorders* (DSM II), which based its classification wherever possible on the psychodynamic understanding of symptom formation. This

Table I. Comparison of DSM II and III Diagnosis Terms for the Neuroses

DSM II	DSM III
Anxiety Neurosis	Panic disorder Generalized anxiety disorder (both are subcategories of Anxiety Disorders)
Phobic Neurosis	Agoraphobia with or without panic attacks Social phobia Simple phobia (all are subcategories of Anxiety Disorders)
Obsessive Compulsive Neurosis	Obsessive compulsive disorder (a subcategory of Anxiety Disorders)

Depressive Neurosis	Major depression with melancholia
	Dysthymic disorder
	  (both are subcategories of Affective
	  Disorders)
	Adjustment disorder with depressed Mood
	  (a subcategory of Adjustment Disorder)

Hysterical Neurosis
  Conversion Type
	Conversion disorder (or Hysterical disorder,
	  conversion type)
	Psychogenic pain disorder
	  (both are subcategories of Somatiform
	  Disorders)

Dissociative Type	Psychogenic amnesia
	Psychogenic fugue
	Multiple personality
	  (all are subcategories of Dissociative
	  Disorders)

Neurasthenic Neurosis
  (Neurasthenia)
	Dysthymic disorder
	  (a subcategory of Affective Disorders)

Depersonalization Neurosis	Depersonalization disorder (or
	  Depersonalization neurosis)
	  (a subcategory of Dissociative Disorders)

Hypochondriacal Neurosis
  (Hypochondriasis)
	Hypochondriasis (or Hypochondriacal
	  neurosis)
	Somatization disorder
	  (both are subcategories of Somatiform
	  Disorders)

has recently been superseded by the third edition (1980) (DSM III), which has made major changes and rearrangements in the diagnostic scheme, using a more empirical, syndromatic approach to the categorization of mental disorders. Although the new scheme has major advantages for clincans dealing with psychotic disorders, in the view of many the abandonment of the traditional classification of the neuroses leads to confusion and overlooks much of the psychological knowledge of their etiology that has been gained during nearly a century of clinical investigation. The terms used here are still retained in the *International Classification of Diseases—9*, and have a greater simplicity and practical utility for the general physician than the scheme proposed by DSM III. Table I shows the comparable diagnostic categories of DSM II and DSM III.

Anxiety Neurosis

Anxiety, one of the most universal of human experiences, is a symptom in most mental disorders. It is the central and characteristic feature of the anxiety neurosis, and occurs in an acute and chronic state.

Acute anxiety can be one of the most painful feelings to which human beings are subject, and when it rises to the intensity of a **panic attack,** is totally disorganizing to the individual's capacity to function. Predominant in the panic attack are a variety of somatic symptoms that result from a massive activation of the autonomic nervous system. Cardiac symptoms are often paramount, with tachycardia, palpitations, and precordial pain that is sharp and sticking in nature. They are frequently accompanied by a sense of breathlessness and air hunger, sweating, and generalized muscular trembling. The patient may also feel urinary or fecal urgency. Central, and perhaps most characteristic of the panic attack, is an inner feeling of horrible dread or a sense of indescribable doom, which the patient cannot specify further except to comment that he feels as if he were going to pass out or to die. The sense of air hunger may cause the patient to hyperventilate, which produces a respiratory alkalosis with the resultant additional symptoms of stiffness, numbness, and tingling in the extremities. These added hyperventilation attacks often significantly compound the patient's despair and terror.

Panic attacks may occur with varying degrees of frequency, ranging from only a few over a period of weeks or months, to the rapid sequence of a large number within a few hours. They may last from a few seconds to several minutes, and generally leave the patient exhausted, apprehensive and demoralized. The attacks usually seem to "appear out of the blue"; and the patient can associate them with no specific event or stimulus: They are "free-floating."

In most cases, the acute attacks arise against a background of chronic anxiety. The latter consists of symptoms that are similar to those of the panic attack, but of lesser intensity—tremulousness, sweating, palpitations, occasional precordial pains, "butterflies" in the stomach, and a general, continuous sense of apprehension that does not have the overwhelming, disorganizing intensity of acute panic. Chronic anxiety is more common than panic attacks, and may be found in many patients who give no history of such attacks. It should also be noted that some patients will complain spontaneously of only one or two of the somatic manifestations. In such cases, a careful history will generally reveal the psychological component of anxiety as well as milder forms of the other somatic symptoms.

Symptoms similar to those of anxiety neurosis may be found in a number of somatic diseases. Two in particular are of practical importance in the differential diagnosis. Hyperthyroidism may have many elements of similarity, and a careful history, examination, and (when indicated) appropriate laboratory tests, should be performed to rule out the possibility of thyroid disorder in patients complaining of anxiety. The cardiac manifestations and chest pain often found in panic attacks may be mistaken for a myocardial infarction. The differential diagnosis may be difficult in the early phases, but the ultimate evidence of myocardial damage in a heart attack will suffice to make a definitive diagnosis. Physicians perhaps err more frequently in not considering the possibility of panic attacks in patients who have acute symptoms with no discernible evidence of cardiac damage, than in overlooking true cardiac disease.

As is the case in all the neuroses, the **treatment** of anxiety neurosis may be long and difficult. Recent clinical experience, however, has shown that further **acute pain attacks often may be dramatically controlled by the use of tricyclic antidepressants or MAO inhibitors.** The relief thus afforded from highly disabling symptoms is a major first step in the patient's recovery. It not only allows him to function in daily life, but enables him to make more effective use of **psychotherapy, which is an essential element in the overall plan of management** for most such individuals.

Central to the psychotherapeutic process is the careful and extended listening to the patient's associations, to determine the basis for the anxiety, which, as has been pointed out, is usually hidden from the patient's awareness. The concern of the physician reflected in his listening and interested attitude is in itself helpful and fosters the positive therapeutic alliance central to the doctor–patient relationship. In the course of this therapeutic dialogue, one can often discover important factors in the production of the patient's symptoms—factors composed both of external anxiety-provoking situations and relationships, and of frightening inner impulses, fantasies, and emotions aroused by the external stimulus. Careful exploration of these factors, and the subsequent airing, elaboration, and understanding of them often bring about lasting psychological changes that attenuate or remove the conflicts that formerly led to anxiety.

Patients suffering from chronic anxiety without panic attacks will often find their symptoms significantly lessened through psychotherapy alone. If, however, the patient has a low tolerance for the symptoms, the **adjunctive use of "minor tranquilizers,"** such as diazepam or chlordiazepoxide, or of propanolol may help to make him more comfortable and functional as psychotherapy continues. Similarly, many individuals can be taught the techniques of systematic relaxation, which help to reverse the sympathetic nervous system excitation and discharge that is immediately responsible for many of the physical manifestations of anxiety. Finally, when anxiety is complicated by hyperventilation, the symptoms resulting from this can often be ameliorated by a simple explanation of the mechanism of symptom production and the use of rebreathing into a paper bag to counteract the excessive loss of CO_2.

Phobic Neurosis

Anxiety is a prominent feature of the phobic neurosis. But unlike its characteristic free-floating state in the anxiety neurosis, in the patient with phobic neurosis it is specifically attached to certain objects, situations or functions. By avoiding these phobic objects and situations the individual is able to prevent the painful experience of anxiety, but in so doing is often markedly restricted in his freedom of activity. It should especially be noted that the **phobia is an irrational fear of an object or situation in which there is, at most, negligible danger.** The patient is aware of this, but knowledge of that fact does not help him to escape the anxiety released by the phobic stimulus.

Phobias fall into three main categories: (1) phobias of function; (2) simple phobias; and (3) phobias of situations. The **phobias of function** are probably the least common, and are seen mainly as a fear of blushing or a fear of eating in public. **Simple phobias** are relatively frequent and involve a wide variety of objects, especially animals such as snakes and spiders. Generally speaking simple phobias cause little in the way of disability since the objects may be avoided with little inconvenience. An important exception in modern life is the *fear of flying*. Many people experience mild to moderate anxiety over air travel but are able to overcome their aversion when flying is necessary. For a significant number, however, the anxiety is sufficient to prevent them from flying at all—a significant handicap for those whose work requires frequent travel and long journeys.

The commonest and most troublesome of the **phobias of situation** is *agoraphobia*. Traditionally the term has been used to refer to a fear of crossing open spaces; but it more properly means a fear of public places where crowds congregate (e.g., in theaters, public transportation, or churches). As a result, the patient often refuses to venture far from the security of his home because of a mounting sense of anxiety the farther he gets from such shelter. Often the anxiety is alleviated if the patient is accompanied by a special person (a spouse, for example); and in the company of that obligatory companion his sphere of activities is broadened. At best, however, the agoraphobic's movements are markedly curtailed; and at worst he may be as totally confined at home as a person with a severely crippling physical illness. Often the onset of agoraphobia is heralded by the sudden occurrence of a panic attack while the patient is somewhere in public. From that point on, he fears the recurrence of the terrifying panic (that is, he develops anticipatory anxiety); and to avoid this recurrence, he increasingly limits his range of activities.

Psychotherapy has been the traditional approach to the treatment of the phobic neurosis and is often helpful in disclosing and reducing the intensity of the psychological conflicts underlying the surface symptoms. Clinical experience has shown, however, that despite the alteration of these underlying factors, the symptoms themselves frequently persist and specific symptomatic treatment is indicated. In patients with agoraphobia **the use of tricyclics and MAO inhibitors** will, as mentioned earlier, often control the outbreak of panic attacks. Despite this, the anticipatory anxiety (the fear of having panic attacks) may persist, and the patient's activities remain seriously circumscribed. In such cases, the addition of the techniques of **behavior therapy** may prove effective in mobilizing the patient to return to an active, unrestricted life. Similarly, behavior therapy may be successful in removing simple phobias. The basic maneuvers in this treatment approach are twofold: (1) requiring the patient to confront the phobic stimulus and to experience the associated anxiety; and (2) the employment of measures that simultaneously help to keep the anxiety at a tolerable level. Finally it should be pointed out that when the patient feels able to conquer his phobia, he experiences a feeling of increased self-esteem and self-confidence, and a sense of freedom to engage in previously interdicted activities that, in addition to symptom removal, are in themselves significant factors in a positive therapeutic outcome.

Obsessive–Compulsive Neurosis

Although anxiety is a component of this disorder, its relation to the specific manifestations is different. In the phobic neurosis, as indicated, the anxiety is associated with a feared external object or situation that can be avoided; in the obsessive–compulsive neurosis the anxiety is attached to internally arising thoughts and impulses that cannot be escaped by avoidance mechanisms. In the phobic neurosis the patient is afraid of being passively harmed by the external environment, whereas in obsessive–compulsive disorders he fears actively doing harm to others around him.

There are two basic components to the obsessive–compulsive neurosis: obsessions and compulsions. **The obsession is a thought that involuntarily obtrudes** itself insistently and repetitively on the patient's consciousness. (Often that one has done something harmful or disgraceful.) **A compulsion is an involuntary impulse to action;** when the patient actually carries out the impulse it is called a compulsive act. Obsessions and compulsions are characterized by the following features: (1) they force themselves on the patient's attention against his will; (2) the patient feels compelled to fight against the intrusions, but is generally only transiently successful in controlling them; (3) they are utterly irrational and unrealistic, a fact of which the patient is aware; and (4) they are generally accompanied by considerable anxiety. Anxiety may become particularly severe when the patient attempts to control the carrying out of his compulsive acts. It should further be noted that compulsive acts are often secondary to obsessional ideas. A patient, for example, had the obsessional thought, "My father will die," every time he turned off a light. To prevent his father's death, he felt compelled to touch the light switch and say to himself, "I take back that thought." He fully recognized the absurdity of both the thought and the ritual touching compulsion aimed at preventing the thought from being translated into reality. Despite this, he was so overwhelmed with anxiety, if he failed to carry out the compulsion, that he was compelled to do so in spite of himself. This example reveals a further characteristic of obsessive–compulsive phenomena—the magical quality of the thought processes involved.

Obsessive–compulsive neurosis ranges in severity from states in which the patient suffers from occasional mild obsessional ideas and compulsive acts that cause him little inconvenience, to conditions in which the greater part of his waking life is occupied with compulsive rituals (such as incessant handwashing to prevent the feared spreading of infection) that keep him from leading any semblance of a useful, normal, productive life. **Patients with the milder forms of obsessive–compulsive neurosis are often helped by psychotherapy.** In many cases this may be provided by the patient's primary physician; the support and reassurance that the patient gains from the relationship with an understanding doctor is sufficient either to remove his symptoms or to keep them at a tolerable level. If the patient fails to respond to such supportive measures in a matter of weeks, he should be referred to a psychiatrist for further evaluation and possible psychotherapy. **Fortunately, the more severe and disabling form of this neurosis is un-**

common, since the symptoms are then generally stubbornly unresponsive to any kind of treatment measures. Some therapeutic successes,
however, have been achieved through the behavioral techniques of
reciprocal inhibition, aversion therapy, and response prevention—a
technique whereby the patient is forcibly prevented from carrying out
his protective compulsive actions with a consequent flooding of anxiety
that ultimately leads to its extinction.

Depressive Neurosis

Like anxiety, depression is a ubiquitous human experience. Whereas
anxiety is a fearful anticipation of trouble to come, depression is a reaction to painful difficulties that have already occurred, most commonly
the loss of a valued person, object, or situation.

Depression is not in itself pathological. Indeed, it would be abnormal
not to feel depressed in the face of the loss of a significant personal
relationship. If, however, the feeling of depression is excessively profound or long lasting given a relatively minor stimulus, and if it is
accompanied by a variety of other characteristic symptoms, especially
serious suicidal thoughts, it should be considered pathological.

Central to depression, as the term implies, is an inner sense of sadness,
emptiness, and often despair, accompanied by a loss of interest in one's
customary pursuits and in people to whom one is ordinarily close. Fatigue, lassitude, and irritability along with a degree of insomnia may be
present, but the presence of severe disturbances in body functions, such
as marked insomnia, anorexia, and weight loss, strongly suggests that
the disorder falls into the category of an "endogenous" depression in
which neurochemical and other biological disturbances play a central
role. The potential for suicide in such patients is a significant complicating factor. Similarly, the evidence of hallucinations, delusions,
and marked self-destructive tendencies are not found in simple neurotic
depressions.

Of particular importance for the nonpsychiatrist is the fact that depressed patients may present themselves with a variety of, often poorly
described, physical complaints—vague aches and pains, malaise, and
minor organ dysfunctions or apparent exacerbations of long-standing
physical ailments whose symptoms are ordinarily tolerated without great
distress when the patient is not depressed. Such patients may not complain of depression, but on a careful history searching for evidence of
precipitating losses and the characteristic signs and symptoms of mild
depression, the diagnosis can often be readily made. In history taking,
the physician should also make a careful assessment of the patient's
suicidal potential.

Neurotic depression generally responds to the support and comfort

to be found in the relationship with an understanding physician. The opportunity to talk to a sympathetic listener about precipitating losses can have a beneficial effect, and the clarification the doctor can provide about the expected course of the illness and any physical symptoms worrying the patient is helpfully reassuring. A mild hypnotic (e.g., Dalmane) may be prescribed if sleeplessness is a problem, but ordinarily antidepressant drugs are neither indicated nor necessary. Indeed, in patients experiencing depression as a reaction to the loss of a significant relationship, it is necessary to experience a certain amount of emotional pain and discomfort in order to proceed through the normal evolution and dissipation of grief. Medication that significantly retards or suppresses such normal processes is contraindicated. **Antidepressant medication is, however, specifically indicated for those patients with the somatic manifestations that indicate the presence of a biological depression (and for those with serious suicidal ideas).** Such patients should be referred for psychiatric evaluation and treatment.

Hysteria

Hysteria is hoary with age. It was known to the Greeks, who described and named it. It has been recognized as an illness ever since, through a long and checkered history whose evolution is not finished yet.

Hysteria is divided into two major forms: (1) *conversion hysteria,* and (2) *dissociative hysteria.* The distinction is made on the basis of the symptoms. Those of conversion hysteria affect primarily somatic functions, while those of dissociative hysteria are manifested in disturbances in mental functions. However, the separation is not an absolute one, for many patients combine symptoms from both categories, and the quality of marked hypnotizability is shared equally by patients with each form.

Conversion hysteria is characterized by a variety of somatic symptoms affecting primarily the sensory–motor system. The motor symptoms are those of paralyses, contractions, and abnormal movements. Sensory symptoms involve all modalities, the most common being anesthesias, hyperasthesias, and paresthesias; blindness, deafness, and anosmia occur less frequently. It is characteristic that neurological examination shows no evidence of localized lesions in the major neuroanatomical systems. Anesthesias and paralyses do not occur in the distribution of either central or peripheral neural pathways; but the form of the symptom is determined by the subjective image of the body. A hysterical paralysis of an arm, for example, will appear as total paralysis and loss of sensation from the shoulder-girdle out to the periphery—clearly delineating the common definition and body-image of an arm. It is furthermore important for the nonpsychiatrist to recognize that **hysterical symptoms may mimic those of physical illness.** This is particularly the case when the patient has lost a close relative and, through a process of identification, develops the symptoms of the illness that led to the relative's death. Or the patient may repeat a symptom pattern from a previous physical disorder of his own.

In **dissociative hysteria** one finds disturbances in consciousness and identity, or both. The commonest and simplest form is **amnesia**, wherein the patient loses the ability to recall events in his past life for a period of time extending from a few hours to several months. Try as he will, the patient cannot bring back to consciousness anything that has happened during this period, although occasionally fragmentary bits of memory return in the form of ego-alien hallucinations (usually visual) or in dreams.

In amnesia the patient may lose his identity, but this is usually transient, and most amnesic patients retain a sense of being the same person throughout a life span that is punctuated by amnesic gaps in his memory. In **fugue states,** disturbance in identity is central. Typically, an individual will drop out of sight, leaving his home, family, and job to become a missing person. Usually he travels far away from his customary abode, and for a period lasting up to months he lives a new life, with a new name, new sense of identity, new job, interests, friends, and pursuits. Then suddenly he "comes to," and often with a feeling of anxiety wonders where he is and how he got there. Now his "old self," he returns to home and family, but with a complete amnesia for the events that have occurred during the period of fugue.

Multiple personality, though the rarest form of dissociative hysteria, is clearly the most fascinating. It is so uncommon as to be of little practical importance for the general physician. Those who are interested will find a number of long case histories in the literature, which often read like novels.

One important fact about all three forms of dissociative hysteria is that **the amnesia is not absolute.** Indeed, in certain states, particularly that induced by hypnosis, all the memories can be recovered. Furthermore, all of the symptoms of both conversion and dissociative hysteria can be produced by hypnotic procedures, a fact that reflects the abnormal propensity of hysterical patients to dissociate or split off certain mental contents and functions from conscious control—whether the dissociation occurs spontaneously or under the influence of hypnosis. Dissociation, in other words, appears to be a phenomenon central to all forms of hysteria.

The term **Briquet's syndrome** (or **somatization disorder**) has recently been proposed to designate a special group of patients, usually women, who are not uncommonly seen in general medical practice. Such individuals may have symptoms that fall into the category of hysterical sensory–motor phenomena described above; these are, however, overshadowed by a wide variety of other somatic symptoms, commonly pain, that mimic the whole spectrum of somatic illnesses. Symptoms referable to the abdomen and generative organs are particularly common, and have in the past led to much unwarranted pelvic surgery (e.g., hysterectomies for removal of "ovarian cysts"). Patients in this group, furthermore, manifest both hysterical and borderline personality characteristics (see below) that complicate the doctor–patient relationship and the clinical management.

The incidence of hysterical symptoms is not easily determined, since there are presumably a number of patients who, in the face of environmental stress, develop single, isolated symptoms whose treatment by an understanding and supportive primary physician leads to the rapid disappearance of their complaints. **Patients with multiple and persistent hysterical symptoms, including those with Briquet's syndrome, should be referred for psychiatric evaluation. Their treatment is often difficult.** Some patients respond to insight psychotherapy or to a variety of hypnotic techniques. Because of the possible complications, hypnosis should ordinarily not be used by the general physician. In general, hysterical patients run a chronic course and require extended care and emotional support. The primary physician can play an important role in this regard, ideally in concert with a psychiatric consultant to whom the physician can turn when complications arise in either symptoms or behavior.

Neurasthenia, Depersonalization, and Hypochondriasis

Little need to be said about these disorders since they are uncommon in pure form. **Neurasthenia** is characterized by excessive fatigue, and is often merely a manifestation of depression. In **depersonalization,** the patient loses a sense of the reality of himself as a person, and, by extension, of the world around him. The symptom may occur alone, but is commonly found in depression, phobic states, and some forms of schizophrenia.

Hypochondriasis has a history as venerable as hysteria. The term is commonly and wrongly used to refer to patients who have a variety of bodily complaints for which the physician can find no somatic basis; more often than not, careful history will reveal that such complaints are the somatic manifestation of depression, anxiety, or hysteria for which specific treatments may be helpful. In its restricted and proper sense, hypochondriasis refers to a rare condition in which the patient presents what are often bizarre symptoms with a conviction that he has a serious medical illness—a conviction that remains unshaken by medical evidence and reassurance to the contrary. The conviction may reach the proportions of a delusion, and as such is often a manifestation of schizophrenia or psychotic depression. The treatment of uncomplicated hypochondriasis is difficult at best. Reassurance to both the patient and his family may provide a supportive therapeutic environment that enables the patient to tolerate his symptoms and to carry on with his every day life and functions. The primary physician should avoid performing repeated and unnecessary examinations and treatments that will heighten the patient's preoccupation with his somatic symptoms.

Personality Disorders

Although the different neuroses are often associated with specific personality types, the latter more frequently occur accompanied by few, if any, overt neurotic symptoms. There have been many schemes over the centuries for classifying personalities, and none is or has been entirely satisfactory or definitive. This should not be surprising if one recognizes that an individual's personality is made up of a variety of patterns of behavior, attitudes, and traits whose combinations are nearly infinite, and which, like the subtle differences in the human face, stamp each individual as a unique person. Rather the wonder is that one is able to find enough in the way of similarities in a group of human beings to establish reasonably distinct categories of personality. **A distinction should be made between personality types and personality disorders.** All human beings have character traits that comprise their personalities. Perhaps most of us exhibit characteristic patterns of behavior and relationships that can generally be categorized as hysterical or obsessional, as these are defined below. Such patterns are not necessarily abnormal or pathological, although they may affect how we react to intercurrent illness and how we relate to those caring for us when we are sick. It is necessary, therefore, for the physician to be conversant with common personality types and their effect on the response to illness.

In some individuals, personality traits achieve a degree of exaggeration and psychopathology that warrant classifying them as personality disorders. In such instances the behavior patterns often bring the individual to medical attention and may require treatment directed at the characterological disturbances themselves. In what follows, only the more common and well-established personality types and disorders will be briefly described. The reader who is interested may consult the appropriate suggested additional readings.

Hysterical Character

Although the features of the hysterical character are usually described as occurring in women, they may be found in men as well. The person with hysterical character traits is colorful, emotional, given to histrionics and exaggeration, and likes to be the center of attention. In giving a history of illness, the patient is frequently dramatic in his description of symptoms or the course of illness, and one is often hard put to discern what is fact or fancy, or to determine the true seriousness and severity of the complaints. Such patients are often seductive in their behavior with physicians of the opposite sex and tend to be exhibitionistic, revealing more of their bodies than is necessary for the requirement of the physical examination, or dressing in such a way that reveals their physical attributes in a manner inappropriate to the sickroom. Finally, individuals with a hysterical character are frequently manipulative and manage to get their own way through fits of temper, threats of suicide, or by otherwise playing on the guilt of others around them. The term hysterical character is often used with pejorative overtones; and it is true that individuals with such traits frequently arouse dislike and anger in others. It must be remembered, however, that such behavior often arises out of a marked sense of inferiority and diffidence, and is aimed at forcing the needed reassuring attention and concern of other people.

Obsessional Character

The obsessional character is in many ways the obverse of the hysterical. Where the latter is emotional, lively, and flamboyant, the obsessional person is measured in his approach, intellectual, often pedantic; he is cautious, logical, and conservative, where the hysterical person is imaginative, even creative. There is a degree of rigidity and inflexibility in the obsessional individual; he is formal in manner, stiff, and reserved in his relationships, and concerned with method and order. He is often stubborn and tenacious in his ideas, but frequently finds it hard to make simple, direct statements without qualifying clauses and reservations, lest he be caught out in an inaccuracy of fact or logic. He is punctual and precise in his dealings with others, is frequently parsimonious if not outright stingy, and sets great store by scrupulous honesty and moral principles. These characteristics, it should be noted, while they may make the obsessional person difficult to deal with, at the same time ensure his conscientiousness and reliability in his work and relationships.

Passive–Aggressive Character

These individuals may show many of the features of the obsessional character. In addition, however, one observes a curious pattern of behavior in regard to aggressiveness. The passive–aggressive person finds it difficult to be openly assertive in making demands on others or in refusing to comply with demands on him from other people. He resists not by directly saying "no," but by quietly, passively failing to comply with requirements imposed on him. He may consistently come late to appointments (often with a seemingly good excuse), fail to make deadlines, "forget" to take medicines regularly, or may in other ways subtly sabotage a treatment program. Seemingly compliant and obedient on the surface, his behavior shows an underlying, indirectly expressed defiance of authority. He lives, in other words, by the principle of acts of omission rather than commission.

Dependent Personality

As the name implies, such individuals are markedly dependent on others for support, help, reassurance, advice, guidance, and direction. They appear unable to make decisions for themselves and leave the determination of their behavior and lives up to others. In a medical situation, they are often unduly incapacitated by illness, and use their symptoms and complaints as a means of getting other people to administer to their wants or as an excuse for avoiding responsibilities and duties. They consult the doctor frequently for the smallest complaint, and often will try to push the doctor to take charge of all aspects of their lives and relationships.

Counter-dependent Personality

Individuals with counter-dependent personality traits are almost the exact obverse of those manifesting a dependent personality. In their behavior and relationships they appear to be constantly trying to prove to themselves and others that they are strong, active, effective, self-sufficient, and capable. They cannot tolerate the role of being a patient or being incapacitated, and will often ignore the increasingly insistent signs and symptoms of serious illness, failing to seek medical help until they are literally physically unable to carry on. Careful psychological exploration reveals a marked underlying tendency toward dependence that the individual cannot accept, and that he hides from himself by patterns of behavior that are totally the opposite from the submerged passive-dependent needs—hence the term **counter**-dependent. It should be recognized that these traits, even though they may have a psychological defensive function, are at the same time a potential asset to a sick person when he does get into medical hands. They provide a strong motivation to return to health and activity as soon as he is physically able. Counter-dependent behavior should therefore be respected by the physician and not viewed merely as stubbornness or a foolhardy disregard of serious illness. When properly understood and managed, such patients can be helped to accept the degree of temporary passivity required by medical treatment without losing their impetus to return to health, activity, and a life of self-sufficient, self-directed responsibility.

Antisocial Personality

Fortunately, persons with antisocial personality characteristics are uncommon, for they can be seriously disruptive to human relationships and the social fabric. On initial contact, such individuals appear to be strong, effective, and self-confident. There is a charm and persuasiveness about them that is often captivating and endearing. Although their apparent warmth is infectious and their seeming sincerity is convincing, the briefest of relationships with them soon reveals their total unreliability. They say one thing and do another; they make solemn promises one minute and break them the next; they convince the unwary of the seriousness of their resolves, purpose, and goals only to veer off moments later in a totally opposite direction. They are the "con-men" of the world; and their evident dishonesty and their lack of resolution and credibility is so destructive and frustrating to others that they have earned the opprobrious epithet of "psychopathic personality" in previous diagnostic classifications. Since such persons are incapable of remaining in a lasting relationship, therapeutic or otherwise, it has been difficult to obtain sufficient information about their psychological functioning to provide extensive understanding of their psychopathology. It is evident, however, that they lack the basic capacity for continuity in their desires, emotions, drives, and relationships. What they quite fervently and sincerely feel and believe at one moment is gone at the next, and the individual goes off abruptly on another tack, which he momentarily pursues with equal sincerity and intensity until once again his capricious inner wind changes. One cannot really get the full flavor of their behavior short of exposing himself to the vagaries of the antisocial personality. He can, however, gain a considerable understanding of the nature of their personality disturbances from the skillful descriptions that have been provided by a handful of sensitive authors.

Borderline Personality

In recent years there has been a great deal of interest in describing, defining, and understanding a group of patients who have come increasingly to form a large part of psychiatric practice—the so-called borderline personality. These personality disturbances are frequently accompanied by a wide variety of neurotic symptoms, and the transient emergence of psychotic symptoms as well. The latter has led to the use of the adjective *borderline* to indicate that such patients, developmentally, characterologically, and symptomatically, fall in a gray area between clear-cut psychotic and neurotic syndromes. The reader who is interested in the complexity of their psychopathology and the attempts to classify them into subtypes should consult the writings of investigators who have made extensive studies of these patients. Suffice it to say here that such individuals manifest serious personality defects in two major areas: (1) their capacity to relate to others at the most basic level of human trust, and (2) a major flaw in their sense of self (their identity), and a related inability to see other people as they really are in all their richness and complexity of character.

The ego deficits in patients with borderline personality disorders stem in part from painful and deforming experiences with others (usually the parents) during the earliest formative period of their personality development. This leaves them with deep dependency needs for support and nurturance from others, accompanied by an ineluctable dread of being hurt and abandoned by those from whom they seek gratification. As a result, their relationships are characterized by a reaching out to others countered by a retraction and withdrawal into themselves. At the same time, by an internal process of "splitting", they tend to see others in black-and-white terms, as all good and giving or all bad and depriving; they are unable to recognize the other person as having a rich fabric of both good and bad traits that characterize human beings. As a consequence, borderline individuals initially reach out for help to a person seen as unrealistically perfect and strong, only to discover flaws and weaknesses that convince them they will not obtain the support they want and need, which they interpret as a total rejection and abandonment. In reaction, they retreat, filled with a rage that is often murderous in intensity, and the formerly idealized person is seen now as utterly uncaring and evil. This process is compounded by the fact that their sense of identity, self-worth, and self-esteem depends on the maintenance of a sustaining relationship. When it is ruptured by the patient's own withdrawal in the face of a sensed rejection, his self-esteem is drastically lowered to a point of despair; and his sense of identity as a person in his own right is compromised, often to the point of a temporary psychotic fragmentation.

The effect of these abnormalities can be readily seen in the course of the doctor–patient relationship. Initially the doctor may be idealized as a powerful, healing, nurturing, and sustaining figure. Inevitably, however, the tide will turn, and the doctor will be viewed as the devil incarnate. He will then find himself the butt of all the rage and fury the patient can muster—a fury that may lead to torrents of verbal abuse, rarely even physical assults. At the same time, the patient will often attempt to manipulate the doctor into providing the help and care that he so desperately needs by entreaties, and by playing on the doctor's guilt with accusations of callousness and cruelty, often accompanied by threats of or actual attempts at suicide. It is important to recognize that throughout these storms the patient has little or no ability to control himself, nor does he have any distance on his behavior or recognition of its utter irrationality. His feelings and his perception of the doctor are experienced by him as being utterly real; and he is totally absorbed in them to the exclusion of any other point of view. It should particularly be noted that when overcome by their pathological rage, such patients often abruptly terminate their relationship with their doctor and consult a new physician; in some this leads to an extended series of abortive medical contacts: "doctor shopping." The understanding management of the patient's rage may hold him in a continued therapeutic relationship, but the physician should not blame himself unduly if he is unsuccessful. The treatment of such patients is exceedingly difficult, and poses problems for which there are not as yet ready solutions.

Therapy of the Personality Disorders

The treatment of personality disorders is often long and difficult. **The approach has generally been that of psychotherapy;** and numerous patients have been helped to achieve a more satisfying life, especially with psychoanalysis, through gaining insight into the psychopathological factors lying behind their disturbed behavior and relationships. At the same time, it must be recognized that the forms of psychotherapy which involve the achievement of insight into unconscious motivations are often not particularly effective with many of the more serious personality disorders.

To be successful, **insight psychotherapy** requires a degree of ego strength that is lacking in many patients with personality disorders. The capacity for insight, the ability to tolerate anxiety, depression, and frustration, the potential to make meaningful and lasting human relationships, motivation to change one's behavior and pattern of living—all are considered by many psychotherapists to be prerequisites for entering into insight psychotherapy. As can be seen readily from the foregoing, in many patients it is just these ego functions that are either absent or severely defective. Accordingly, some clinicians feel that insight therapy is generally contraindicated in patients with such severe disturbances, and that the clinical approach should be that of **supportive psychotherapy,** involving the control of behavior through the setting of limits, advice, exhortation, and the general emotional support to be gained from a relationship with a strong, confident, compassionate, and caring physician.

Recently a number of clinical investigators, especially those working with patients with borderline character disorders, have suggested that, with appropriate modifications, **psychoanalytic techniques** can be useful. The first task, in their view, is to deal with the patient's fundamental difficulty in making relationships, through a long period of providing a human environment in the therapeutic situation whereby the patient may develop the capacity for basic trust and strengthen his sense of identity and self-esteem. Once this has been accomplished, then the patient will be capable of a more extensive exploration of his psychopathology through the more traditional analytic techniques of the insight psychotherapies. The ultimate effectiveness of this therapeutic approach remains to be seen, but meanwhile the work of modern investigators employing these therapeutic measures is of great interest and is vastly increasing our knowledge of the clinical and developmental disturbances that constitute the severe personality disorders.

Additional Readings

Neuroses

Clinical Psychopathology. Edited by Balis JV, Wurmser L, McDaniel E. Boston, Butterworth, 1978, Section 3, pp 207–330

Diagnostic and Statistical Manual of Mental Disorders, 2nd ed. (DSM II). Washington, DC, American Psychiatric Association, 1968

Diagnostic and Statistical Manual of Mental Disorders, 3rd ed. (DSM III). Washington, DC, American Psychiatric Association, 1980

Nemiah JC: Depressive neurosis, in Comprehensive Textbook of Psychiatry II. Edited by Freedman A, Kaplan H, Sadock B. Baltimore, Williams & Wilkins, 1975, Chapter 21, pp 1255–1264

Nemiah JC: Neurotic Disorders, in Comprehensive Textbook of Psychiatry, 3rd ed. Edited by Kaplan H, Freedman A, Sadock B. Baltimore, Williams & Wilkins, 1980, Chapter 21, pp 1481–1517, 1525–1561

Personality Disorders

Clinical Psychopathology. Edited by Balis JV, Wurmser L, McDaniel E. Boston, Butterworth, 1978, Section 4, pp 333–367

Cleckley H: The Mask of Sanity. St. Louis, Mosby, 1950

Diagnostic and Statistical Manual of Mental Disorders, 2nd ed. (DSM II). Washington, DC, American Psychiatric Association, 1968

Diagnostic and Statistical Manual of Mental Disorders, 3rd ed. (DSM III). Washington, DC, American Psychiatric Association, 1980

Gunderson JG, Kolb JE: Discriminating features of borderline patients. Am J Psychiatry 135:792–796, 1978

Kernberg O: Borderline Conditions and Pathological Narcissism. New York, Aronson, 1975

Stanton AH: Personality disorders, in The Harvard Guide to Modern Psychiatry. Edited by Nicholi AM. Cambridge, MA, Harvard University Press, 1978

Vaillant GE, Perry JC: Personality Disorders, in Comprehensive Textbook of Psychiatry, 3rd ed. Edited by Kaplan H, Freedman A, Sadock B. Baltimore, Williams & Wilkins, 1980, Chapter 22, pp 1562–1590

Chapter 9

Stress, Situational Maladjustment, and Grief

Eugene A. Kaplan

Stress

Stress is ubiquitous; it is an inevitable concomitant of lived experience. Stress can be biological (illness, trauma, starvation), psychological (death of a loved one, divorce, job loss), or social (war, poverty, persecution). What varies tremendously is the individual's capacity to cope or adapt.

In modern times, the term stress has had two broad usages. In one, stress refers to the events and traumas individuals may find disturbing or injurious. In the other, it refers to the individual's response to these disturbing stimuli. Hans Selye's work focused on the response-oriented concept: "Stress is the nonspecific response of the body to any demand made on it" (1956, p 1). More recently, others (e.g., Holmes and Rahe's "Schedule of Recent Life Experiences,") have focused on the precipitants or stimuli which people often find stressful. Another, even more comprehensive approach defines stress as the discomfort generated by the interaction between an individual and his environment. Both stressors and responses are important to the individual and the physician.

Life Stresses (Stressors)

Some life stresses are universal, i.e., they can occur in any culture and at any point in the life cycle and still be stressful. Serious physical illness and injury are good examples of such stresses. Others are more phase-specific; they occur at particular points in an individual's life cycle, or in a particular social or cultural context. Infants are particularly vulnerable to the stress of separation from the mothering figure; young children to leaving home and entering school; adolescents to the vicissitudes of first sexual encounters, medical students to the National Board Exams, senior citizens to retirement, etc. Needless to say, not all such events are necessarily traumatic. People vary greatly in their vulnerability. Even good experiences can be stressful, e.g., promotions at work, winning the lottery or getting married can all produce a stress response, even if perceived by the individual in positive terms.

Holmes and Rahe have proposed an ordering of life events which trigger stress and require some readjustment or adaptation. In this scale, the death of a spouse is seen as the most traumatic or stressful life event for the majority of adults and used as the index against which to measure stressors. Other highly stressful life events include divorce, death of a close relative, being fired, and retirement. Middle-range events include trouble with in-laws, children leaving home, and change in financial state or work responsibilities. Less stressful events include change in residence or school, vacations, and minor violations of the law.

Of equal importance to the specifics of the scale, is the notion that such **life events can be viewed cumulatively;** i.e., a series of otherwise manageable life stresses may overload the individual and produce a maladaptive response: The "straw that breaks the camel's back." Individuals with high total life change scores on such a scale are more vulnerable to stress responses or illnesses than individuals with low scores.

Of special concern to physicians, is **physical illness as a stressor as well as the result of stress.** From our point of view, a patient's illness is a challenge; a problem to be solved—in as competent and humane a way as possible. From the patient's viewpoint, illness is stressful quite apart from, or in addition to, the specifics of the particular condition. Pain, suffering, and disability, or the fear of any of these, are stressful. Fears of death and dying are frequently invoked by even mild illnesses. In the face of serious illness, such as heart disease or cancer, these fears can be intense. Treatment itself can be stressful: surgery is the paradigm of this, both in terms of the physical demands made upon the body, and the emotional demands of a procedure which may be unconsciously perceived as an assault or threat to life.

Thus a physician assessing a patient's illness needs to be aware of the stress that the experience of illness and treatment causes, for that particular patient, as well as the particular disease process itself.

The Stress Response

Selye developed the concept of a "general adaptation response," the notion that there is a generalized, nonspecific, and defensive organismic response to stimuli, regardless of their specific nature. This consists of three phases: an alarm stage, in which the body initially perceives the stressor and begins to react; a resistance stage, in which adaptive mechanisms are actively in play; and an exhaustion stage, which comes about if the defenses and adaptive mechanisms are inadequate, or if the stressor lasts too long. While the concept of this syndrome initially was conceived primarily in physiological terms, it has since been modified and expanded to include psychological reactions as well.

The **common psychological reactions of acute stress** include anxiety, fear, increased irritability, increased attentiveness to external stimuli, a readiness to fight or flee, rumination, insomnia, restlessness, moodiness, tension, difficulty making decisions, and, in some instances, difficulty concentrating. Later reactions may include fatigue, exhaustion, low self-esteem and depression. Should any of these reactions last too long, be experienced too intensely, or become unduly disabling, we call such phenomena *situational reactions* or *adjustment disorders*, conditions to be discussed later in this chapter.

The **common physiological reactions** include an increase in the rate and strength of the heartbeat, an increase in the rate and depth of respiration (sometimes leading to the symptoms associated with the hyperventilation syndrome), a redirection of the blood supply from the skin and viscera to the muscles and brain, dilation of the pupils, increased sweating, etc. These changes are initiated and mediated through complex neuroendocrine mechanisms whose end results include an increase in the secretion of epinephrine (and to a lesser degree, norepinephrine), which seems to dominate during the alarm stage of the acute stress reaction, followed by increased production of adrenal–cortical hormones, primarily the glucocorticoids. Other neuroendocrine systems, such as the pituitary–thyroid axis, also may be involved.

It is important to note that **the stress reaction is a total organismic one:** the psychological, physiological, and behavioral responses are indelibly intertwined and interrelated. The physician who understands this, and also understands that some type of stress response is normal and expectable will be in a better position to anticipate, reassure, support and, when necessary, treat the responses.

Posttraumatic Stress Disorder

There is a special syndrome following those psychologically traumatic events above and beyond the range of usual human experience. Such severe stressors as assault, rape, combat, floods, earthquakes, plane crashes, bombing, concentration camps, or multiple losses (e.g., of one's entire family) can produce a profound stress disorder. This posttraumatic stress disorder usually begins with an **acute stage** characterized by severe anxiety, hyperalertness, an exaggerated startle response, difficulty falling asleep, and nightmares, often reliving the traumatic event. Many individuals also experience a dramatic decrease in responsiveness to the outside world, referred to as psychic numbing or emotional anesthesia, shortly after the traumatic event. **Later stages** of the disorder are characterized by sleep disturbances, difficulty concentrating, inhibited social and sexual relationships, guilt about personal survival if others did not, and frequent depression. While these symptoms may begin shortly after the traumatic event—and often continue for many months—they may also emerge months after the stress, or, in some cases, even years later.

The **treatment** of this disorder is complex, and usually should be attempted by a specialist with substantial knowledge of this type of problem. The acute stage usually requires substantial emotional support and the opportunity for catharsis, if the patient is able to talk about the event. It is often necessary to have the patient relive or reexperience the memory of the trauma, in the safety of the relationship with the therapist. This reliving (*abreaction*) is occasionally facilitated by hypnosis or drug assistance (the amytal interview). The purpose is not only to remember but to come to terms with (*work through,*) the problem or trauma. Issues of survival guilt sometimes must be addressed. Continued psychological and emotional support are usually needed for a substantial period of time. Occasionally the use of anxiolytics such as the benzodiaxepines is necessary and helpful.

Situational Maladjustment (Adjustment Disorders)

Far more common than the posttraumatic stress disorders, are a group of **maladaptive reactions** to various psychosocial stressors. The maladaptive nature of these stress responses is indicated whenever symptoms occur substantially in excess of the normal or expected reaction to the stressor, either in duration or intensity, or the individual becomes significantly impaired or disabled, in his social function. Usually these reactions begin shortly after the stress is experienced, most often within 3 months.

These maladjustments can occur in reaction to the previously mentioned life stresses (e.g., divorce, marital difficulty, business failure, loss of job, retirement, desertion by spouse or lover, increased responsibilities or workload, etc.). The **severity of the response is not necessarily related to the severity of the stressor;** adjustment disorders are a function of the particular meaning and intensity of a stress in the context of a particular person's life. Vulnerability varies greatly from individual to individual.

Types of Adjustment Disorder

There are five common types of adjustment disorder. These include disorders characterized by **anxiety,** where the dominant feature involves such symptoms as anxiety, nervousness, or excessive worry; by a **de-**

pressed mood, with dominant symptoms of sadness, tearfulness, and hopelessness; by a **work inhibition,** with a major decrease in work or academic functioning; by **withdrawal,** in which the individual substantially disengages from social relationships; and those characterized by a **disturbance in conduct** (acting out), often including such behaviors as reckless driving, getting into fights, or drinking too much. Many involve some combination of these. A mixture of anxiety, depression, and work inhibition is very common.

Treatment Considerations

Treatment generally involves three steps or processes. The first is the **identification of the life stress** to which the individual is reacting. While many patients are aware of the stressor, a surprising number are not, or fail to make the connection between significant life events and their subsequent subjective distress. The second step is **ventilation and reflection,** an opportunity to share not only the stressful experience, but the feelings associated with it. The third involves **working through,** or coming to terms with the problem. Often this involves finding new or substitute solutions to the problem which was threatening to overwhelm the individual.

If the uncomfortable feelings associated with these stresses are too intense or too painful, certain medications may be helpful if used **sparingly** and for **brief** periods. A benzodiazepine (e.g., Librium, Valium) in small or moderate doses often can reduce anxiety to more tolerable levels; tricyclic antidepressants (e.g., Elavil, Tofranil) are sometimes useful in reducing or alleviating even mild to moderate depressions. However, if the patient can manage reasonably well without medication, it is preferable to do so. Even Valium can be habituating; and to learn to deal with life's problems without mood-altering medications is far preferable in the long run.

Many physicians can be very helpful with the less complex adjustment disorders if they are skillful and able to take the time it requires to help a patient identify and discuss a problem. More complex problems should be referred to the psychiatrist.

Grief

Grief is the natural response to the death of a loved one. The need to grieve is a fundamental human characteristic, in which the pain of a major personal loss is both expressed and, to some degree, discharged. The ways in which grief is experienced and expressed are functions of the nature and strength of an individual's attachment to another; personality style; the religious or cultural background from which one comes; and the opportunity to grieve. It is no accident that the three major religious traditions of the West, regardless of their differences, each offer—even encourage—a significant period of mourning; the necessary time to do much of the work of grieving; the support of living friends and relatives; and funeral services and related ceremonies which honor the dead and comfort the living.

Most people turn to their **families and friends** for solace. Usually these are the people who are in the best position to help the grieving individual bear the pain of the loss. Emotional ties of long duration are never more important than at the time of death; they remind the grieving individual of shared experiences and memories, and of important relationships which continue even in the face of immediate loss.

The **clergy** can be especially effective in helping many individuals deal with grief. This is an integral part of the clergy's work and training, coupled with psychological sensitivity, a knowledge of the family, and a religious–cultural tradition within which to express and guide the grieving process. Physicians can enlist this major resource when trying to be of help to those grieving families for whom religious ties are significant.

The **physician** has three major tasks in helping families with grief. The first involves helping families **anticipate** a loss, whenever possible. Anticipation can, at best, give people an opportunity to prepare for a death and begin to come to terms with a loss which seems to be inevitable. While no one totally works through a death in advance of the actual experience, alerting if it is done in a language and style appropriate to the needs and mood of the family, can be very helpful.

The second task centers around the immediate **announcement of death.** It is usually a physician who announces death to a family—just as, in a happier context, it is a physician who announces birth. Unfortunately, there is a temptation to report the bad news and then escape as soon as possible. While this may protect the physician from his own feelings—including the feeling of defeat—it shortchanges the family at a time when support and comfort would be most helpful. Death is, of course, hard on physicians as well as families; often the physician himself has enjoyed a long and friendly relationship with his patient. He too may be in mourning—but responsibility to the family must transcend that feeling, especially the tendency to disengage as quickly as possible.

It is the physician's continued presence and quiet support, more than the specifics of what is said, that matter most. Sometimes just sitting quietly with a family, giving them an opportunity to ventilate their grief—and occasionally their anger—can be very helpful. Reassurance that all was done that could be, and that the patient was kept as comfortable as possible, may help ease the family's minds about the final illness and death. Sometimes merely quietly answering the family's questions is best.

Even the occasional family member who becomes "hysterical" at the news of death will usually calm down after 5 to 10 minutes in the presence of a strong, kind, and supportive physician. Often the offer of a cup of coffee or some equivalent will help; rarely, a mild sedative is needed. Eventually the physician can disengage; the family needs time to be alone and express its grief in private, and the physician may also need time to work through his own feelings, as well as continue with other responsibilities.

The third task for the physician is to be aware of and alert to, *pathological grief*, which lasts **too long,** is experienced **too intensely,** or **becomes disabling through excessive guilt, depression, or rarely, suicidal intent.** Pathological grief is a relatively uncommon extension or complication of normal grief. Such examples as Queen Victoria's deeply mourning Prince Albert for 20 years, to the neglect of her duties, remind us that no one is immune to this.

A resonable standard for grief varies from individual to individual and culture to culture. Most people are able to return to their jobs and obligations within a month or two, if not sooner, even after a very significant loss. Of course, considerable sadness lasts for many months, and may linger for a year or more. Mourning which lasts more than many months or continues unabated in intensity, can be considered pathological.

As with adjustment disorders, pathological grief may require therapeutic intervention. Sometimes a physician's gentle encouragement—even permission—to disengage from excessive mourning is all that is needed. A redirection of interests from the dead to the living, even if couched in terms of responsibility (rather than spontaneously achieved) may ultimately set the stage for full return to function. However, there are times when neither the physician's nor the clergy's interventions are effective. This usually signals a problem that goes deeper than the loss itself, however important; and which requires referral for psychotherapy.

Rarer are instances in which an individual fails entirely to grieve an important loss, even privately. Apart from the adaptive strain, this unresolved grief sits, lurking just below the surface, not unlike a walled-off abscess ready to burst open later after a minor injury. Some of the severe depressive situational maladjustments represent such **delayed grief reactions** triggered by a subsequent loss that itself may be trivial. These too are likely to require psychotherapeutic intervention.

Additional Readings

Cox T: Stress. Baltimore, University Park Press, 1979

Diagnostic and Statistical Manual of Mental Disorders, 3rd ed. (DSM III). Washington, DC, American Psychiatric Association, 1980

Holmes TH, Rahe RH: The Social Readjustment Rating Scale. J Psychosomatic
  Res 11: 213–218, 1967

Lazarus RS: Psychological Stress and the Coping Process. New York, McGraw-
  Hill, 1966

Parkes CM: Bereavement: Studies of Grief in Adult Life. London, Tavistock,
  1972

Selye H: The Stress of Life. New York, McGraw-Hill, 1956

Simons R, Pardes H: Understanding Human Behavior in Health and Illness.
  Baltimore, Williams & Wilkins, 1977, Chapters 27, 36; pp 295–304, 378–386

PART III

AGE-RELATED DISORDERS

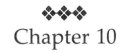

Chapter 10

Evaluation and Treatment of Children

David A. Waller and Leon Eisenberg

Physicians normally feel apprehensive about evaluating children for emotional and behavioral disorders, and with good reason. We are never quite sure in advance what will be the most productive way to conduct an interview with a particular child or adolescent; and there is the lurking fear that "he won't talk to me." We sense that we are in less control of the situation than is usually the case in our practice of medicine. Furthermore, it may be difficult to distinguish the disturbance that should be refered for the specialized care of a child psychiatrist from the more common behavioral upset that may constitute a vicissitude of normal development, and respond to simpler measures. The task of evaluating children is made somewhat easier, however, by the fact that a great deal of helpful information can be obtained from the child's parents and teachers.

Information about the Child

Interview with Parents

Our objective is to identify and evaluate children's problems in a way that meshes with the parents' own view of their child and supports their self-esteem. It is good practice to **give parents the opportunity to talk about any behavioral concerns they may have, even during medical visits and routine checkups.** Though not voiced as a "chief complaint," these concerns may have in part prompted the visit, at least in part. If a behavioral symptom comes to light in this way, the parents should first be asked their own views about it and whether we can be helpful to them in attempting to sort it out. Parents may minimize or even be unaware of a problem we think may be serious; conversely, they may be overly concerned and need reassurance. A good rule of thumb is to avoid taking a position that is in major opposition to the parents'. Fortunately, a period of time is usually available during which additional appointments can be scheduled, additional data gathered, and, hopefully, some agreement reached as to the nature of the problem and best course of action.

An accurate, unambiguous, and detailed **description of the problem behavior** should be obtained, including when it first began, its frequency and intensity; and, if the child is brought for a behavior problem, why that help is being sought **now**. Commonly, the problem has been present for some time. The event that precipitated referral is almost always revealing. Furthermore, it is important to ask: Has help of any kind (psychiatric or other) been sought in the past? Was it helpful? If not, what were the hopes and expectations that were not met? History tends to repeat itself in these matters, unless we are careful to explore the reasons for the repeated consultation. Permission can usually be obtained to talk with prior helpgivers.

Careful attention should be given to any relevant **physical disorder.** The child's medical history, starting with the pregnancy and neonatal course, is important: because serious illness is a significant stress on family life; because disease can impair the child's development; and because brain dysfunction can be an important contributing factor to psychiatric difficulty. Psychiatric disorders occur at a much higher rate among children who are neurologically impaired in comparison to classroom controls. Family history may be relevant—especially a history of psychiatric illness, both because it may provide clues to relative risk of similar difficulty in the child and because it may generate unwarranted fears in the parent about the inevitability of a similar outcome for the patient. It is critical to recognize when a child's behavior problems are a consequence of treatable brain disease. Deteriorating school performance, neurologic signs and symptoms, episodic outbursts of behavior, and alterations in awareness are some of the ways **brain syndromes** may present.

Psychosocial stressors comprise another important class of information. These include illness or death of a parent, sibling, or other close family member; parental separation, divorce, or remarriage; economic crises; moves; and school failure. More difficult to ascertain may be distress resulting from inability of a family to provide for the emotional needs of a particular child. This can result from the combination of adverse circumstances and dissonance between the parents' personalities and that child's temperament. The physician who knows the family from past contact may feel uncomfortable in exploring family interactions as they pertain to the child's problem. This can be accomplished more successfully if the focus is on what the family may be able to do to help the situation, as opposed to what they may have done to contribute to it. Families are likely to feel less threatened by working on these problems with their family physician or pediatrician rather than a psychiatrist.

Finally, the child's **adaptive functioning** should be assessed. Can he work, love, and play? School performance commensurate with ability; age-appropriate meaningful friendships; and the ability to enjoy oneself are some of the markers of mental health. Conversely, subjective distress and/or impairment in one or more important areas of functioning defines mental disorder. We are interested in the current level of adaptive functioning, the highest level in the past year (which may have prognostic significance), and how the child negotiated important developmental landmarks like toilet training, the birth of a sibling, or the beginning of school. We sometimes forget to inquire about the child's strengths, but these too are important if we are to have a picture of the child as a unique human being. In what situations, and with what strategies, has he demonstrated the ability to cope well? What are his special interests or hobbies? How is this child especially likable?

School Information

If the child goes to school, the history is not complete without information from the teacher. Parents should be asked to sign a consent form releasing school information to the physician, with the explanation that this is routine. Teachers are likely to be more objective than parents, and have the advantage of seeing the child in a setting with other children of the same age. Important areas like cognitive functioning and interactions with adults and other children are observed directly. In the case of school complaints about the child, telephone conversations with key individuals may provide the richest history and make the case come alive. They also provide the opportunity for the physician to express interest and concern for the distress the child is causing.

Summary

Every child is a part of a system consisting of parents and family, teacher and classmates, and neighborhood friends. Our goal is to determine what persons are registering a "chief complaint," what is the nature of their concern, and what are the factors in the child's environment and in the child which may contribute vulnerability to dysfunction. The registering of a complaint by a member of the child's network does not necessarily mean there is something wrong with the child. Parents may, without realizing it, be seeking help for themselves, or even for another child at home whose problem is too upsetting to address. Conversely, a very disturbed child may not be identified as needing help if his behavior is not upsetting someone else. Examination of the child will help clarify some of these issues.

Examination of the Child

The **goals for the physician in the initial session(s)** with the child are: (1) to help the child feel at ease with the physician; (2) to form an opinion as to the nature and severity of the child's problem; and (3) to make a decision as to how urgently further evaluation and help is needed, and what form this should take. We turn over to the child, with certain limits, the allotted time, materials, and even ourselves, so that the child can fashion out of these resources a session that will say something meaningful about that child's way of behaving, thinking, and feeling.

That this technique often is initially anxiety-provoking for the physician is expectable, given the lack of teaching in medical school and residency. It sometimes requires an exhausting amount of flexibility, patience, and ingenuity. Since an endless variety of novel circumstances can occur, it is helpful to have a colleague with whom one can discuss the inevitable challenges that arise.

The actual methods used to accomplish these goals depend to a large extent on the age of the child. For purposes of discussion, children can be grouped by age.

Infants and Toddlers

If behavioral problems are involved, an appointment should be scheduled when both parents can be present. This rule applies generally to psychiatric evaluations of children. Provided the physician is flexible about times, it is reasonable to expect both parents to arrange to be present, given sufficient notice. The **infant or toddler is seen in the company of parents.** A few age-appropriate toys should be in the room for the child to use as he likes during the initial part of the session, while the physician obtains the history. This allows the child to feel more at ease in the presence of a stranger. It also permits the physician to observe the child's interactions with his parents, his response to a new situation, and his use of the materials at hand.

We are interested in getting a feel for whether the child is at age level for the pertinent **developmental milestones** for his age-group. These can be divided, as in the Denver Developmental Screening Test, into social, language, gross-motor, and fine-motor skills. Most children can sit with some support by 6 months and walk with help by 1 year. Playing simple games like "peek-a-boo" and "pat-a-cake" are an important milestone of social development at about 10 months. By 1 year most children say a couple of words, and by 2 use a couple of elementary sentences or phrases. These landmarks are outlined in more detail in Lewis's (1971) manual of child development. The limits of normal have wide variation.

If there appear to be developmental lags, either across the board or primarily in one area, consultation should be obtained from a developmental psychologist, for precise assessment. While we do not want to create undue anxiety in parents, referral to a specialist can be explained as simply reflecting how difficult exact evaluation is in this age-group, rather than implying the child necessarily has a serious problem. It may make an enormous difference to the child if a problem can be detected early and managed appropriately.

In this age group, the "psychological" problem of greatest concern is the child who doesn't relate well to people. At the extreme is the autistic child who literally reacts to people as though they were inanimate objects. (The word psychological is placed in quotation marks because autism and other serious behavioral deviations in young children are likely to have a strong constitutional or organic component.) Remediable medical conditions may present with a picture resembling a primary behavioral disturbance: visual or hearing difficulties; metabolic disorders like hypothyroidism or phenylketonuria; lead poisoning; child abuse with subdural hematoma. When the physician is satisfied that medical diseases have been excluded, the child with autistic behavior or other severe behavioral deviation should be referred to a child psychiatrist who specializes in work with very young children.

Preschool Children (3 to 6 Years)

During this period children normally master self-care skills like dressing and undressing and become quite competent at communicating with adults and other children. Experiences like nursery school or play groups allow the child to become comfortable even though his parents are not at hand, and the ability to play cooperatively is an important social milestone. **If a vulnerability to learning dysfunction is suspected, it should be evaluated carefully by a psychologist.** While many difficulties improve with maturation, the child may benefit greatly from special-needs programs which give support and assistance in areas where extra help is required, and the physician may be instrumental in guiding parents to the appropriate resource for evaluation and intervention.

Children this age comprehend what is being said about them. To preserve the child's self-esteem and encourage forthrightness on the part of the parents, **separate interviews should be conducted.** Indeed, it may be advisable for the parents to arrange for the child to remain at home when they first come to discuss their child's behavior problem in detail. The attempt to see the child alone may or may not be successful, depending in part on whether the child has experienced time away from the parents. One takes note of the child's response to the "separation" experience of going into the doctor's office without parents. If the child balks and clings to a parent, an attempt is made both to reassure the child as well as to bring about a successful separation eventually. One may, for example, show the child where the parent will be waiting while the child is with the physician, or have the parent briefly accompany the child into the doctor's office, or have the parent wait in an adjoining (but separate) room.

Preschoolers generally have very active imaginations and like to play. It's easier to get to know the child if there are a few toys available for the child to become involved with. We observe the child's physical appearance and how he relates to us; his predominant mood state and other feelings that he expresses; his general level of intelligence and any thoughts or subjects he seems preoccupied with; his behavior during the session; and his attention span. Interspersing questions about the activity at hand and about areas more directly related to the problem behavior may provide useful information, as well as permitting observations of the child's speech. Throughout, the physician should try to convey friendliness and genuine interest in the child.

The child psychiatrist often uses symbolic play as a diagnostic technique for these children. When a "pretend house" (dollhouse) outfitted with figures representing the important people in children's lives is turned over to the child, what follows is often a remarkable symbolic display of what is most on the child's mind—what he feels most sad, angry, or frightened about. The physician with a particular interest in evaluating children of this age may want to familiarize himself with this method.

Elementary School Children

Behavior problems occur frequently in this age-group, especially in boys. **These children tend to be among the most difficult to get to know,** however, because they are self-controlled and not inclined to reveal thoughts and feelings. Chatting over a board game that does not require the child's total attention may break the ice and provide for a useful exchange of information. A question-and-answer approach can be employed, but it should be noted that the child probably has a defensive bias against the questioning adult. The teacher who asks questions does so to test for information; the parent who says, "Why did you do that?" doesn't really want to know why. Thus, to be successful, questions for the child must be nonjudgmental, and must convey interest and the physician's desire to share with the child what the child has been thinking and feeling.

The physician may **begin by asking the child what he has been told about the visit.** If the child has no information, or denies having any, the doctor can state in general terms what the concerns are and whom they come from, adding that he is interested in understanding things from the child's point of view. It is helpful to approach threatening material from safer ground. Thus, discussions about things the child likes to do, and is good at, should precede talking about a problem area like school. Interest in hearing about things that make the child feel happy should precede questions about sad or frightening material, or things that make the child angry. As the child talks, it helps to point out the feelings being expressed, with the reassurance that all children—indeed all people—have the same kinds of feelings.

A simple but useful technique is to ask the child what **three wishes** he would make if a good fairy were suddenly to appear. The things wished for often reveal how the child would like life to be changed. One can also offer, as a bonus to the thoughtful child, a special wish for mother and for father. Asking a child to **draw a picture** of a boy and of a girl permits a rough estimation of mental age by assessing the detailed characteristics of the drawing; the picture may also be psychologically revealing by indicating feelings about the self and awareness (or lack of it) of sex differences. A drawing of "your family doing something" is helpful in eliciting the child's sense of position in the family and the feeling tone of family interaction.

The physician must be alert to the need for **prompt intervention in the presence of psychotic or suicidal ideation.** The child who reports bizarre ideas should be questioned to see if those ideas are considered to be real or imaginary. In a child who seems depressed, one should not hesitate to explore potential suicidal trends. One can point out that sad children sometimes "even wish they weren't alive," and ask if the patient ever feels that way. If he has, has he ever reached the point of having a plan to hurt himself? If a child is not suicidal, asking about it does not give him the idea. The danger is in failing to elicit the information when the child is feeling truly desperate. Idiosyncratic thinking that forms the basis for action and/or suicidal preoccupation may indicate the need for prompt hospitalization, depending upon the estimate of risk.

Another indication for psychiatric referral and hospitalization is the child who is unable to separate from home in order to attend school, and with whom attempts at outpatient treatment have proved unsuccessful. A chronic medical problem may complicate **school phobia,** but the inability to go to school may be altogether out of proportion to medical needs.

Adolescents

The incidence of severe psychiatric disturbance rises in adolescence.
Psychosis is characterized by the loss of contact with reality. Psychotic
disorders of thought content include *delusions*—fixed false beliefs that
an individual cannot reason about, and which are not part of a cultural
belief system; and *hallucinations*—external sensory perceptions occurring
when no external stimulus is present (hearing voices, for example). The
form or structure of thinking can also be disordered, as in *loose associations,* in which the flow of ideas appears random and disconnected; and
flight of ideas, a characteristic finding in acute mania in which thoughts
go rapidly one to another but are connected in meaning.

Psychosis in adolescence is an acute emergency, and suggests the
possibility of the onset of schizophrenia or manic–depressive disease.
More common as a cause of psychosis in this age group, however, are
organic factors like **drug intoxication or withdrawal.** These conditions
may be specifically treatable and should be considered especially when
there is alteration in the state of awareness; disorientation; cognitive
deficits; memory loss; or visual, olfactory, or tactile hallucinations. Amphetamine abuse, phencyclidine ("angel dust") intoxication, and herpes
simplex encephalitis are of special interest in that they can all present
with psychosis and a clear sensorium.

Another emergency is the adolescent who is suicidal, who requires
expert consultation, and frequently hospitalization. **Suicide ranks third
as a cause of death in adolescence.** Attempts greatly outnumber completed suicides and are more common in adolescent females, whereas
males more frequently kill themselves. Most are **not** psychotic. It is
helpful to assess intent by comparing the relative risk of the gesture
with the opportunity for rescue that was present. While this risk–rescue
ratio provides an index of the need for hospitalization **every** suicide
attempt in adolescence represents a desperate request for a change in
some aspect of the adolescent's life situation, or relief from an unbearable
feeling, or expresses rage toward a significant person in the adolescent's
social system, usually a parent; it must be taken seriously as a communication of troubled feelings.

Most adolescents with behavioral difficulties are neither psychotic nor
acutely suicidal. The adolescent should be reassured that while there are
problems to be addressed, this does not mean that he is "crazy." The
concerns that have been expressed to the physician can be described to
the patient. **Confidentiality should be offered,** excluding only material
relating to the immediate risk of harming oneself or others. Then an
attempt is made to convince the adolescent to use our services for his
own ends. Are there ways he wishes his life were different? Perhaps
we can be of help.

At a suitable point, **progress in the specific developmental tasks of**

adolescence should be evaluated: separating from family and forming an independent identity; proceeding in education toward an appropriate job or career; and establishing successful relationships with members of the same and opposite sex. Adolescents who appear to need help, but who either deny this or do not want it, present a real quandary. An adolescent is old enough to have a say in such matters, and to attempt to force the issue is merely to reenact the struggle for autonomy that is likely to be going on between the adolescent and his parents. On the other hand, some teenagers hope the physician will care enough about them to keep encouraging them to obtain further help.

Diagnostic Impressions and Treatment Considerations

The physician who has obtained a history as outlined above and who has spent one or two sessions getting acquainted with the child will have at least partial answers to the important questions an evaluation seeks to elucidate. In what ways, and to what degree, is this child dysfunctional, or in distress? What appear to be the important biological, psychological, and social determinants? Does the pattern of behavioral symptoms fit any specific diagnostic entity? [The third edition of the *Diagnostic and Statistical Manual of Mental Disorders* (1980) (DSM III) provides critera for child and adolescent psychiatric conditions.]

How rapidly intervention begins depends, in part, on the degree of upset in the child or in his network of family and school associates. Relevant medical factors must, of course, receive prompt attention. Treatment of children's behavioral difficulties often requires a blending of biologic, psychodynamic, and behavioral models. [These are summarized in volume III of the *Basic Handbook of Child Psychiatry* (1979).] A child with an attention deficit disorder and hyperactivity, for example, might respond to a combination of stimulant medication, counseling of parents and teachers, and psychotherapy to help the child deal with his frustrations and low self-esteem. Whatever role the physician chooses to play in carrying out a specific dimension of the evaluation and treatment process, the principles outlined here should allow the physician to perform an invaluable service to the family by orchestrating the evaluation and management of the child's behavioral problem.

Additional Readings

Basic Handbook of Child Psychiatry. Edited by Noshpitz D. New York, Basic Books, 1979

Diagnostic and Statistical Manual of Mental Disorders, 3rd ed. (DSM III). Washington, DC, American Psychiatric Association, 1980

Lewis M: Clinical Aspects of Child Development. Philadelphia, Lea & Febiger, 1971

Rutter M: Helping Troubled Children. New York, Plenum Press, 1975

Simmons E: Psychiatric Examination of Children. Philadelphia, Lea and Febiger, 1974

Vaughan VC: The Denver Developmental Screening Test, in Nelson's Textbook of Pediatrics. Edited by Vaughan VC, McKay RJ, Behrman RF. Philadelphia, W.B. Saunders, 1979

Yudkin S: Six children with coughs. Lancet 2:561–563, 1971

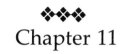

Chapter 11

Common Behavioral Disorders of Childhood

David A. Waller and Leon Eisenberg

Detailed consideration of the more serious psychiatric disorders affecting children and adolescents is inappropriate in this book. Their treatment, or even the unraveling of their differential diagnosis in ambiguous situations, requires the skill of the child psychiatrist. A very brief discussion of the major psychoses is given at the end of this chapter to alert the practitioner to their general features.

There are, however, a number of common conditions about which the primary care physician or general psychiatrist should be thoroughly informed. The recognition and management of the majority of patients with these problems is well within their capacity. It is especially to the former that families turn for advice and help; and their involvement ordinarily is preferable because stigmatization is minimized.

Enuresis

Bedwetting is probably the most common behavioral condition for which help is sought. Most children acquire the capacity for bladder control by age 2 to 3. Somewhat less than 15% fail to do so by 5; and by age 8, less than 7% have more than occasional "accidents." Draft statistics reveal its incidence to be around 2% in males by age 18.

Organic factors are not common. Because urinary infections are more common in enuretics than the general population, although not present in most enuretics, **routine urinalysis is always indicated.** Outflow obstruction, however, is sufficiently rare that **routine exploration of the**

outflow tract is not indicated. Such instrumentation procedures themselves are upsetting to a child and may cause infection.

Twenty to 25% of enuretic children do demonstrate the presence of psychiatric disturbance (particularly those past age 9 and girls). Hence, other signs of disturbance should be sought for, and appropriate referral made. But **enuresis alone should not be considered a psychiatric disorder.** It is best conceptualized as a problem in learning, although a reduced bladder capacity may contribute in some children.

Daytime wetting is much less common than that at night. Less than 2% of 5-year-olds wet during the day as often as once weekly; and less than 1% of 8-year-olds once a month. Its management is the same as nocturnal enuresis. Combined day and night enuresis is more often associated with psychiatric disturbance and with urinary infections.

Treatment

Treatment usually is based on applied learning principles ("behavioral therapy"). Before considering these, it is important to note that **the commonsense approach of nighttime fluid restriction and awakening almost never works.** The doctor who recommends this is likely to impair his credibility when it fails.

One useful approach is the "Star Chart." The parents, with participation of the child, mark each episode of enuresis on a calendar. After a baseline, a gold star is awarded for each dry night, and pasted on the corresponding date with appropriate praise. After a specified number of stars, an agreed-upon reward is supplied. The baseline rate is used to set the target: the child who wets nightly should be rewarded for the first dry night; whereas for the intermittent wetter this is given only after a longer-than-usual dry period. With successive improvement, the requirement for reward is increased stepwise.

Another method focuses on **increasing bladder capacity.** The child is encouraged to defer urination during the day, while increasing fluid intake. Urine volume is measured each time; and praise (and target rewards) given for progressively larger volumes. Although useful, this method involves a major time commitment by the parents.

The *bell and pad device* consists of a buzzer or bell linked to two electrodes implanted in (or placed on) a cotton sheet upon which the child sleeps. Wetting closes the circuit, activating the alarm powered by a dry cell. The noise immediately awakens the child—and the parents. The child then is required to go to the toilet to complete bladder emptying, and then to change the sheets, with parental help as necessary. Success can be achieved within a reasonable time in more than two-thirds of enuretic children. While relapse may occur in as many as a third of these, this can be greatly reduced by increasing bedtime fluid intake (by

500 cc) for several weeks after complete dryness is achieved, before discontinuing the apparatus. The bell and pad is probably the most effective of the reeducation methods, but involves some expense, and may be difficult for a family living in close quarters.

In **all** these methods, the **likelihood of success will be greater if the physician maintains ongoing contact** with the family, to provide support and to encourage consistent and persistent use of the technique. Premature discontinuation is a commmon cause of failure.

Drug treatment is not recommended. Anticholinergics have been used extensively; and amphetamines also have been tried; but neither has proved effective. Imipramine (25 mg in children under 30 kg; 50 mg in larger children) has been used with excellent **initial** effectiveness; and may be tried if other methods have failed, or to obtain a quick short-term result, as when a child is seen a week before going to overnight camp. However, relapse is the usual outcome.

Sleep Disturbances[1]

The doctor must assess complaints of disturbed sleep against developmental norms. The duration, distribution, and stages of sleep are age related. Its average duration is 15 hours at 1 month; 12 hours (plus an hour nap) at 2 years; 11 hours (plus nap) at 4; 10 hours, at 8 to 12; and 9 at adolescence. The newborn rapidly adapts to the day/night cycle; naps are limited to the afternoon by 1 year, and are rarely necessary by 5. The neonate spends 80% of its sleep in the Rapid Eye Movement (REM) stage, later associated with most reported dreams; but by 1 year, this declines to the adult value of 25%.

Isolated episodes of difficulty falling asleep, bad dreams and night terrors, and partial somnambulism are seen in virtually all children. Stress frequently leads to transient disturbances in sleep, which respond readily to parental reassurance. During the second year, the normal child may resist going to sleep because of disinclination to give up activity or attention. Fears at night are common in the 3- or 4-year-old. In each of these, parental response is decisive in determining the subsequent outcome. An overly harsh attitude to normal fears and interests, or too-easy acquiescence to wishes for comfort can prolong otherwise minor, transitory behavior.

Counseling by the physician is the treatment of choice. Most sleep problems are best understood as learned responses, and approached in terms of extinction of these patterns and relearning socially desirable ones. Medication should be limited to situations of acute distress, and

[1]Chapter 16 considers these disorders in adults.

then used only briefly. Tolerance develops rapidly; habituation may occur; and "rebound" insomnia (often with nightmares) follows any prolonged use.

Night terrors and nightmares are more common and benign in children than adults, and less likely to be associated with other signs of psychiatric disturbance.

Night terrors (pavor nocturnus) occur during **non**-REM sleep, accompanied by intense anxiety with autonomic arousal (including tachycardia), vocalization, and poor recall. The child is not fully awake, though the eyes are open. Screaming or crying, and clutching or running away from the parents may occur. Restraint may be required to prevent self-harm.

In contrast, the *nightmare* occurs during REM sleep, like ordinary dreams; and is usually associated with less severe anxiety. Often the child can report the vivid, frightening dream.

The usual prognosis for nightmares and night terrors in children is excellent, with conservative management. Reassurance and comfort are all that is usually required. Recurrent nightmares are an indication for the physician to explore family stress. Persistence suggests the need for more thorough behavioral evaluation. Medication is rarely indicated.

Sleepwalking (somnambulism) also is common in childhood. These episodes occur during deeper non-REM sleep, as with night terrors; and like the latter are associated with poor awareness and recall. Psychopathology is not commonly associated; though this is suggested by later-age onset and persistence. In the absence of psychiatric disorder, sleepwalking disappears or greatly diminishes within a few years. Again, **treatment centers around reassurance.** The child and family should be informed of its benign nature and prognosis. In addition, active measures must be taken to **protect the child from injury:** sleeping on the ground floor, securing doors and windows, etc.

Hypersomnia is uncommon in children and adolescents. Its presence should be taken seriously as an indication for thorough diagnostic workup. Among its causes are brain pathology, the Kleine–Levin syndrome (with bulimia), the Pickwickian syndrome (with obesity and impaired respiration), and significant depression.

Obesity

Obesity is traditionally defined in terms of body weight. But this must be considered in relation to height, sex and body build. Age is another factor: weight tends to underestimate body fat below age 7, and overestimates it in adolescence. Skinfold thickness is a more accurate index. Twenty percent above norms is a good criterion for medical purposes, because excess death rate begins to appear above this figure. Fat children tend to become fat adults; and early-onset obesity is far harder to reverse in adults than that of adult onset. Early attention to the problem may, therefore, have long-term health benefits.

Family factors, both genetic and environmental, are important in etiology. Other known sociocultural factors are social class (lower) and ethnic background. Psychological studies indicate that the meanings of food (e.g., as affection) and of body size itself play a role. There is evidence also that obese people are more sensitive to the temptations of such external cues as the sight, odor, or presence of food, or clock mealtime. Actual **psychopathology occurs only in a minority; and a true physical (metabolic, endocrine) basis is rare.**

Treatment rests on modifying the balance between caloric intake and expenditure. Increasing the patient's level of activity is a valuable, oftneglected approach, though usually reduced intake is also necessary. **The most important factor in success is the motivation of the patient and family.** This involves not merely the wish to lose weight but their willingness to modify well-entrenched, covertly highly valued patterns of eating behavior. The doctor's initial decision, then, is to assess motivation against the degree of overweight (medical necessity). The older the child, the more this must include the child's motivation, as well as the parents'.

Ongoing general psychotherapeutic support is essential, whatever the treatment technique. Caloric restriction is experienced as deprivation, and interference with ongoing routines and food or eating patterns as additional frustration. Both parents and child need support; and the parents need help in supporting the child. Many fat people feel guilty and ashamed of their state, feelings which reinforce eating as a form of substitute satisfaction. If the parents or physician enhance this by criticism, the likely result will be paradoxical. Warm, active support, combined with praise for efforts and rewards for successful weight loss, is far more fruitful. Given the typical slow progress, low rate of treatment success and frequent recurrences, the physician is hard-pressed to maintain patience, much less a positive attitude; yet maintain them he must.

If other signs of psychopathology are present, appropriate treatment directed at the more important overall psychiatric condition is indicated. Often this requires referral. As the disorder improves, so may the weight. But in the usual instance of uncomplicated obesity, psychotherapy alone rarely is successful.

Dietary counseling is important. Basic principles of good nutrition should be taught. For the infant, dietary restriction is contraindicated. Rather, the parents should be counseled on ways to comfort their child other than relying primarily on feeding. For children under 5, the emphasis should be on altering the diet rather than food restriction (e.g., substituting skim for whole milk). In older children, the extent of caloric restriction must be modest enough to ensure that growth is not inhibited: either weight is kept constant or loss is limited to under 0.5 lb per week.

Special diets are not indicated except in the very rare instances where a specific metabolic abnormality is present. Fad diets do not enhance success, and carry the dangers of causing nutritional imbalance.

Drugs are dangerous and ineffective. This includes hormones (e.g., chorionic gonadotrophins) in the absence of a demonstrable endocrinopathy. Induced puberty (itself undesirable) simply converts a fat child to a fat adolescent.

Special summer camps for obese children may be helpful. They enhance motivation and self-confidence, restrict calories, and interrupt entrenched familial eating patterns.

Behavioral modification methods probably are the most generally successful. In these the emphasis is on **eating behavior** rather than caloric restriction, which occurs secondarily. Special training in the details of this method is required, usually necessitating referral to a psychologist, psychiatrist, or pediatrician already expert in its use. A number of the successful commercial weight reduction programs rely heavily on behavioral techniques combined with psychotherapeutic support in a group setting. These may be helpful for adolescents.

"Hyperkinesis" (Attention Deficit Disorder)

Overactivity, distractibility, impulsivity, and labile mood, often accompanied by serious learning difficulties, characterize this syndrome. It occurs in 2 to 4% of school-age children, being four times as common in boys. Complaints of these symptoms require a full and careful behavioral evaluation. A reportedly "hyperactive" child may actually be suffering from an anxiety disorder, temper tantrums, hyperthyroidism, etc. The hyperkinesis is probably more an inappropriateness of behavior in social situations demanding calm, rather than overall increased motor activity. It is less common in one-to-one situations with an adult—including the physician.

The symptom providing the greatest handicap is usually the distractibility, because of its effects on school achievement. Many regard this as the core defect, thus the recent official renaming, *attention deficit disorder*. Because some authorities believe that the syndrome arises from subtle neurological defects, it also has been termed *minimal brain dysfunction* (MBD).

The first step in treatment is to counsel the parents, teachers, etc., about the nature of the syndrome. Notions that the child is "bad" or "stupid" are corrected. Situations in which hyperactivity will prove troublesome are avoided, and sedentary activities encouraged, while outlets for discharging normal "energy" are provided. The school should be assisted in designing a program tailored to the child's specific profile of deficits and assets.

Stimulant drugs (d-amphetamine, methylphenidate) are valuable

for overt symptoms but will not improve learning without an appropriate school program. A drug trial should begin empirically, with the lowest dose. This can be increased slowly to reach a satisfactory response, up to toxicity or maximum dosage. Morning or early afternoon administration is required to prevent insomnia. Medication should be withheld on weekends, holidays, and vacations: its primary purpose is to help school behavior and learning. Height and weight must be monitored because these drugs can impede growth.

Behavior modification techniques have proved valuable also, and may turn out to be as useful as drugs. This requires referral to experts in the use of these techniques with children. (Such experts, unfortunately, are rare.)

School Phobia

This condition is **an inability to attend school because of a persistent unrealistic dread and/or recurrent physical complaints.** The latter include bellyaches, headaches, fatigue, weakness, or other complaints which appear or increase when it is time to go to school. Unless the doctor is alert to this issue of timing, his skills may be taxed by obscure, puzzling symptoms.

The child's inability to separate from home is the core factor. Careful exploration will reveal that almost always **this is mirrored in the parents' difficulty in "letting the child go"** (usually the mother). The parents' conscious wish to have the child attend school motivates medical consultation, despite the coexistent covert overprotectiveness.

Careful diagnosis is crucial. The behavior of child and parents, the timing and variability of symptoms, the identification of sources of anxiety in the family, and the usually adequate academic performance of the child will support the diagnosis. Major psychiatric disorder (autism, depression, retardation, etc.) should be ruled out. Truancy can be differentiated because the truant child, often in academic difficulty, is able to leave home, though he never appears at school or is gone before the day's end. Physical examination will allow the physician a credible basis for informing the family that the disorder is psychological, and reveal the rare instances where physical disease may coexist.

Once diagnosed, **the central approach is prompt return to school. Home teaching is a grave error,** and likely to result in chronic disability. A persistently firm, reassuring attitude on the part of the physician is crucial. In early or mild cases, this usually will suffice. The longer the prior absence from the school, the more complicated is the process of return. Careful prior preparation of parents and school officials is then necessary. The ease of treatment and prognosis is better for elementary school children, for whom separation anxiety is more age appropriate. The problem is greater for older children, and may represent but one part of serious, pervasive psychopathology necessitating referral for treatment. Adolescents often require referral to a psychiatrist expert in working with this age group; behavioral (desensitization) treatment, medication (tricyclic antidepressants), and hospitalization may be required.

Learning Disorders

About 10% of nonretarded school children are said to have difficulty learning in school. There are many potential contributing factors that require diagnostic exploration. Among these are biologic disorders like anemia or petit mal epilepsy; psychologic factors like anxiety or hostility toward an overly demanding parent; and social factors: children in lower socioeconomic classes may be predisposed to school failure in part because of the social situation. Disruptive behavior at school like "clowning" may mask an underlying problem in learning. Conversely, learning difficulty may be associated with an underlying psychiatric disorder like hyperkinesis (attention deficit disorder) or affective illness (depression).

Early detection permits early assessment and intervention, which may prevent more serious problems later. Because the learning process begins with perception, vision and hearing should be carefully screened. An overall IQ assessment by a psychologist experienced in working with children will be helpful in establishing the diagnosis and making the appropriate school choice.

Some of these children will be considered to have a *Learning Disability*. This term refers to a disorder in which the child who is free of physical handicaps or the effects of poverty and cultural disadvantage but is unable to learn adequately despite having normal intelligence. Presumably the learning difficulty arises from subtle dysfunctions in the central nervous system.

The nature of the child's learning process deficit should be defined as specifically as possible, so that an appropriate remedial teaching program can be designed. Complicating emotional factors are almost always present and should be identified and addressed (especially common are problems related to damaged self-esteem); and an effort should be made to recognize and build on the child's special strengths and talents.

Childhood Psychoses

Infantile Psychosis (Autism)

This rare disorder **appears prior to 30 months of age.** It is characterized by extreme avoidance or ignoring social contact, insistence on environmental sameness, stereotyped movements, severe impairment of speech and language or muteness, and markedly uneven intellectual performance. Intelligence may be at any level. Neurological findings usually are noncontributory. No fully effective treatment exists. Some gains can be made by behavioral modification (taught to parents for their use). Drugs may be symptomatically helpful. For children with normal or better IQ, psychotherapy and special schooling are indicated.

Symbiotic Psychosis

This syndrome, also rare, was described by Mahler. Occurring between age **2 and 5 years,** it is manifest by generalized panic reactions with desperate clinging behavior to the mother, along with oddities of behavior or thinking which may resemble autism or schizophrenia. In the absence of a thought disorder like delusions or loose associations (which if present raises the possibility of schizophrenia), these children would now be classified as having a *Childhood-Onset Pervasive Developmental Disorder*, the essential features of which are a profound disturbance in social relations and multiple oddities of behavior, developing after 30 months of age and before 12 years. The long-term prognosis is probably better than that of Infantile Autism.

Disintegrative Psychoses

This term refers to a **heterogeneous group** of rare syndromes, **appearing after age 3** in children with prior normal development. Some cases may later be identifiable as specific neurodegenerative syndromes; others are of unknown cause. The course is inexorably downhill with severe retardation, though survival may be prolonged.

Childhood Schizophrenia

Another rare condition, this is clinically similar to adult disorder, but occurs in children **after age 7.** Its features include autistic withdrawal, disorganization, and peculiarities of thought, blunted or inappropriate affect, delusions, hallucinations, etc. The course is chronic, with periodic acute exacerbations requiring hospitalization. Continuing psychiatric care is required. Neuroleptics may be helpful. Even in the best of instances, only a relatively marginal life in a protected environment (family or institutional) can ordinarily be expected.

Additional Readings

Bruch H: Eating Disorders: Obesity, Anorexia Nervosa and the Person Within. New York, Basic Books, 1973

Childhood Obesity. Edited by Winick M. New York, Wiley, 1975

Eisenberg L: School phobia: A study in the communication of anxiety. Am J Psychiat 114:712–718, 1958

Eisenberg L: The pediatric management of school phobia. J Pediat 55:758–766, 1959

Eisenberg L: The management of the hyperkinetic child. Develop Med Child Neurol 8:593–598, 1966

Eisenberg L: The clinical use of stimulant drugs in children. Pediatrics 49:709–715, 1972

Kales A, Jacobson A, Paulson MJ, et al: Somnambulism: Psychological correlates. Arch Gen Psychiat 14:586–604, 1966

O'Leary KD, Pelham WE, Rosenbaum A, et al: Behavioral treatment of hyperkinetic children. Clin Pediatr 15:510–515, 1976

Pierce C: Enuresis, in Comprehensive Textbook of Psychiatry II. Edited by Freedman AM, Kaplan H, Sadock BJ. Baltimore, Williams & Wilkins, 1975. Chapter 37, pp 2116–2125

Shaffer D: Enuresis, in Child Psychiatry. Edited by Rutter M, Hersov L. Philadelphia, Lippincott, 1977, pp 581–612

Silver L: The minimal brain dysfunction syndrome, in Basic Handbook of Child Psychiatry Volume 2. Edited by Noshpitz JD. New York, Basic Books, 1979, pp 416–439

Stunkard AJ: From explanation to action in psychosomatic medicine: The case of obesity. Psychosom Med 37:195–236, 1975

Webb WB: Length and distribution of sleep and the intrasleep process. Int Psychiatr Clin 7:29–31, 1970

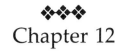

Chapter 12

Geriatric Psychiatry

Gene D. Cohen

Aging is an experience we all obviously share. How one defines "old" is another matter, given frequent discrepancies between chronological age and physical or psychosocial functioning. More for reasons of common reference, social convention, and statistical expediency the 65-and-older group is considered as the geriatric population.

By 1975 in the United States there were over 20 million people (10% of the population) 65 and older; by 2030, 50 million persons will be in this age-group. One must be careful with generalizing about a group of this magnitude. While there are certain common clinical issues, **the approach to the older patient must be individualized,** just as the approach to younger patients is.

Facts and Myths

What is normal aging; and what is illness in later life? The difference between the two is often not obvious. Too many treatable disorders are dismissed as inevitable, irreversible concomitants of the aging process. A wide range of myths, stereotypes, and misinformation interfere with the recognition of symptoms in older persons—many of the same symptoms which would register concern when found in younger adults. Unless clinical problems are perceived as such, a plan for treatment will fail to follow. Some of the big offenders include the following.

Change in Sleep Pattern

When an older person says he has been sleeping less, he is commonly assured that this comes with aging—that it is normal, and not to worry.

Not necessarily so. Although various sleep studies indicate that a reduction in total sleep time occurs in later life, others have not. At best, the change is a group characteristic which does not apply to all individuals; and the reduction which occurs is typically quite gradual. Consequently, **sleep changes should not be taken for granted,** especially if of recent onset. If the older person reports sleeping less recently—not just sleeping less at night because of naps during the day—then an evaluation should be done. Apart from potential medical problems of cardiologic, arthritic, or urologic origin, psychiatric disorders can have sleep changes as hallmark symptoms. Early morning awakening may be an important clue pointing to an underlying depression. Difficulty falling asleep or restless sleep with frequent awakenings may signal anxiety.

Change in Intellectual Functioning

When an older person complains of a change in intellectual functioning those around him too often jump to the hasty conclusion that he's "getting old" or "senile." Extensive research, including longitudinal studies, have shown that older adults who maintain their general health and remain intellectually active in later life show no significant cognitive decline with aging. One study of normal, healthy elderly men done at the National Institute of Mental Health revealed no drop in their average IQ, over a 12-year period.

The point is not that changes fail to take place. Older people do not, for example, react to stimuli as quickly. But vocabulary can increase with aging. The point instead is that noticeable intellectual change should be seen first as a symptom suggesting an underlying problem that may respond to treatment. Such problems could range from hypothyroidism to an insidious pneumonia to depression—to name only a few causes.

Relevant to this is the extent to which **senile dementia is overdiagnosed and misdiagnosed.** Senile dementia is not a part of aging; it is a disease of unknown etiology. Several studies have found that probably less than 5 to 6% of persons over 65 manifest senile dementia. Moreover, many patients with seeming dementia will be found on closer examination to be suffering instead from depression or other nonorganic psychiatric conditions, a condition termed *pseudodementia.*

Talk About Death

Because the elderly have a larger number of acquaintances who have died, talk about death or those dying is understandable. But preoccupation about death, especially dread of it, rather than being normal in later life **may reflect an underlying depression** caused by some loss—loss of a loved one, loss of financial independence, loss of self-esteem.

Interestingly, concern about death is more typical in the middle years when one often first becomes profoundly aware of his mortality. By later life, denial about death once again sets in as a constructive defense mechanism to allow one to continue through life with less anxiety.

Longevity

Some wonder if comprehensive evaluations and treatments are indicated for the elderly since "they do not have much time left." Longevity data, though, can be misleading. While the average life span in America is about 73 years, these figures reflect longevity from birth. **By age 65 one is essentially a survivor, with an average life expectancy of another 17 years** (more for women); at age 75, one has on the average another nine years, and so forth with aging. Clearly, there is ample time for both life and treatment for most elderly people.

Course of Illness

The concept of exacerbation and remission of illness seems less well appreciated with psychiatric than with medical disorders. When someone with diabetes or congestive heart failure has a flare-up, family and physician expect that a remission is likely to follow with proper treatment. An aggravation of a psychiatric disturbance, however, is more likely to be met by others with greater impatience and disappointment or a sense of futility. Such reactions can be magnified when the patient is an older person. The point to keep in mind is that psychiatric, as well as medical disorders, can remit, and can do so in later life as well as earlier.

A corollary of this is that exacerbations in later life must not be overlooked. Moreover, rationalizations like "depression is a part of old age" do not help. In fact, they are dangerous. That **the elderly have the highest rate of suicide of any age-group** speaks to this point. It is at least as risky to downplay psychiatric disturbances with older people as it is with younger ones.

Institutionalization

Part of the reason that health professionals have such a skewed image of the elderly stems from the nature of clinical training. Most of their exposure to older persons has been to a hospitalized, sick, and debilitated population. But most older people are definitely not in transit to an institution. Indeed, at any point in time **only 5% of the over-65 age-group are institutionalized.** Ninety-five percent of people over 65— nearly 20 million—are in the community, not in institutions. The clinical picture of the 95% should not be confused with that of the invalided 5%.

Evaluating the Older Patient

More with the older patient than perhaps any other, the medical maxim to "address the total patient, with attention to the interplay of the biomedical, the psychological, and the social" should be heeded. If the basic approach of a thorough history and workup used for all patients is followed with the elderly, the practitioner rarely will go wrong in identifying existing problems. But, again, since the interplay of physical and psychosocial factors is often more marked with the elderly, **a comprehensive assessment is essential.** Several patterns reflecting this interplay may emerge:

1. Psychiatric problems with medical sequellae

   Example: depression → dehydration, poor nutrition, anemia due to anorexia and poor intake

2. Medical problems with psychiatric sequellae

   Example: hearing loss → paranoid thinking
   Note: Hearing loss occurs to varying extents in 30% of the elderly. The consequent sensory deprivation makes one more at risk for developing paranoid ideation, even delusions.

3. Psychiatric problems aggravating concurrent medical problems

   Example: Cardiac disease plus depression → congestive heart failure

   Explanation: The depressed individual may lose his will to survive and his motivation to take his cardiac medication (passive suicidal behavior).

4. Medical problems aggravated by lack of adequate psychosocial supports

   Example: Multiple medical problems plus living alone → poor management of problems and pursuit of follow-up care
   Note: One out of three older women and one out of seven older men live alone.

Mental Status

One of the most challenging parts of the differential diagnostic workup of an older patient is determining whether a mental problem is "organic" or "nonorganic" (functional), or a combination of the two. A range of laboratory and special tests in addition to sophisticated psychological testing can be utilized. But for purposes of quick and immediate tentative assessment, two basic approaches can be followed:

THE GENERAL MENTAL STATUS EXAMINATION

Within the general mental status examination (described in Chapter 2), five areas are specifically relevant to evaluating organicity. These, and the changes which may occur, are:

1. Orientation to time (date), place, and/or one's own identity may be altered.
2. Recent memories (yesterday's meals, activities, repeating six or seven numbers) and remote memory can both be affected. Problems with recent memory are often more apparent.
3. Intellectual functioning may be impaired, where difficulty with calculation, interpretation (of proverbs), comprehension, and general information can be detected.
4. Judgment may be impaired.
5. Affect may be labile or shallow.

THE BRIEF MENTAL STATUS QUESTIONNAIRE (MSQ)[1]

Question	Mental Status Component
1. Where are we now?	Orientation to place
2. Where is this place located?	Orientation to place
3. What day of the month is it?	Orientation to time
4. What month is it?	Orientation to time
5. What year is it?	Orientation to time
6. How old are you?	Memory: recent
7. When is your birthday?	Memory: recent–remote
8. What year were you born?	Memory: remote
9. Who is President of the United States?	General information; recent memory
10. Who was the President before him?	General information; remote memory

In scoring this ten-item questionnaire, 0 to 2 errors indicate absent to mild organic brain syndrome; 3 to 5, mild to moderate; 6 to 8, moderate to severe; 9 or 10, severe. Clearly this test has limitations when subtle changes are being explored, and is not necessarily conclusive, but it has a useful quick screening value.

[1]See Kahn RL, Goldfarb AI, Pollack M, Peck A: Brief objective measures for the determination of mental status in the aged. Am J Psychiatry 117:326–328, 1960.

Psychiatric Problems in Later Life

Any of the psychiatric disorders that trouble younger patients can be found in the older person. Studies indicate that the incidence of significant psychiatric symptomatology in old age is in the range of 18 to 25%. For the most part, the major psychiatric syndromes of the elderly include transient situational disturbances, affective disorders, anxiety states, hypochondriacal disorders, paranoid reactions, and "alcoholism," as well as organic brain syndromes.

Depression

The most common psychiatric problem in later life is depression. It is also one of the most varied in terms of its different causes and diverse forms of presentation, such as the following:

CLASSICAL FORM
Feelings of sadness, guilt, worthlessness, hopelessness, fatigue, and anorexia, as well as signs of tearfulness, withdrawing behavior, weight loss, irritability, anger, agitation, and sleep disturbance.

MULTIPLE SOMATIC COMPLAINTS
Complaints of gastrointestinal problems, diffuse aches and pains, as well as general hypochondriacal concerns may be symbolic cries for help signaling an underlying depression.

VAGUE PHYSIOLOGICAL DECLINE
Unexplained physical deterioration may have depression at its roots, reflecting a giving-up feeling as in the example about congestive heart failure and passive suicidal behavior mentioned earlier.

PSEUDODEMENTIA
This atypical form of depression is too often misdiagnosed as dementia. Its symptoms may include patchy memory impairment, defective orientation, and vague or inappropriate answers to questions, associated at times with bizarre delusions and a sense of a mild depression. This apparent dementia disappears with proper treatment of the depression. As many as 15% of elderly depressives may manifest their disorder with pseudodementia.

DRUG-INDUCED DEPRESSIONS
Reserpine, though less used today in the treatment of hypertension (one of the most prevalent disorders of the elderly) can cause depression as a side effect in perhaps 15% of those on higher dosages. The depression

may begin as soon as 1 week or as late as 14 months after starting this medication. It should be noted also that alpha-methyl-dopa and some other antihypertensives, and many other medications, can cause depression in a small percentage of patients.

Psychiatric Treatment in Later Life

A number of general and specific points should be made about psychiatric treatment for older people:

Psychiatric problems in later life, like those of earlier adulthood, **respond to a range of treatment approaches**—"talking-about-problems therapy" (individual, group, family therapy), pharmacotherapy, improved family and social supports, and so forth. The elderly, too, commonly respond to brief therapy.

Symptoms of dementia demand an aggressive differential diagnostic workup, since rather than senile dementia, they may be signaling a number of treatable disorders ranging from acute brain syndromes to depression (pseudodementia). It should also be kept in mind that psychogenic and organic problems can coexist and that either or both may respond to proper treatment with overall improvement in the clinical state of the patient. A case in point is the stroke patient whose reactive depression makes him look more impaired and keeps him from effectively participating in a rehabilitation program. Another example is the patient with organic brain syndrome who has secondary symptoms such as delusions or hallucinations, both of which may be alleviated with appropriate medication.

When a psychiatric disturbance is manifested through multiple somatic complaints the appropriate intervention is not a confrontation or interpretation of the symptoms, since these are defenses, but a willingness to help the patient and to explore the psychological and social stresses that are precipitating the complaints.

Sometimes the only way pseudodementia can be diagnosed is after trial treatment, such as with antidepressant drugs, followed by clinical improvement.

With psychotropic drug use in the elderly, "start low and go slow." Because of altered metabolism with aging, lower dosages are generally required to reach both effective and toxic blood levels in older patients. Potential side effects must be understood and carefully monitored, particularly hypotensive and anticholinergic symptoms. The latter can seriously aggravate glaucoma and urologic difficulties associated with prostatic hypertrophy. Moreover, with the greater use of medications by the elderly, **one must always be alert to drug–drug interactions.** For example, blockade of the so-called norepinephrine pump by the tricyclic antidepressants and certain phenothiazines prevents accumulation of the antihypertensive guanethidine and thereby antagonizes its hypotensive effect.

As a final point, it should be emphasized that the interplay of physical and psychosocial factors, just as in the diagnostic workup of the older adult, must be rigorously addressed in the overall treatment plan.

Additional Readings

Butler RN, Lewis MI: Aging and Mental Health. St. Louis, Mosby, 1973

Cohen GD: Approach to the geriatric patient. Med Clin N Am 61(4):855–866, 1977

Fann WE: Pharmacology in older depressed patients. J Gerontology 31:304–310, 1976

Human Aging II: An Eleven-year Follow-up Biomedical and Behavioral Study. Edited by Granick S, Patterson RD. Washington, DC, Department of Health, Education, and Welfare, Publication HSM-71-9037, 1971

Kahn RL, Goldfarb AI, Pollack M, Peck A: Brief objective measures for the determination of mental status in the aged. Am J Psychiatry 117:326–328, 1960

Mental Illness in Later Life. Edited by Busse EW, Pfeiffer E. Washington, DC, American Psychiatric Association, 1973

Roth M: The psychiatric disorders of later life. Psychiatr Ann [Vol. 6]:57–101, 1976

PART IV

EMERGENCY STATES

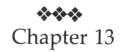

Chapter 13

Evaluation of the Emergency Patient:
Suicide, Violence, and Panic

Magnus Lakovics

Definitions of psychiatric emergencies range all the way from statements such as, "any patient with a psychiatric condition who appears in an emergency room" to "any patient whose psychiatric condition is an immediate threat to life and limb." This reflects more on the actual range of psychiatric patients seen in emergency settings than on an absolute definition of a psychiatric emergency. Regardless of definition, patients present as emergencies with disorders ranging from mild adjustment reactions to acute psychoses. Most emergency states in medicine are characterized by their acuteness, the degree of threat to life, the need for accurate, rapid diagnostic assessment and treatment to offset sequelae or complications from delay (e.g., lacerations). Psychiatric emergency states share these characteristics. But, in addition, they sometimes entail distortions and disorders of consciousness and thought which may result in violence to self and others.

Pitfalls

Requests for emergency medical services in current American practice have become more common and less emergent. Ambulatory patients frequently use the emergency room (E.R.) when their physician or clinic simply are not available. Patients often find it easier to reach a physician on emergency call or to make an unscheduled emergency visit to the doctor's office or clinic, rather than waiting until the morning or for an appointment days or weeks later. As emergency medicine grows as a specialty, expanded emergency services will develop still further. With this, the expectation that emergencies will be only the most "acute" (interesting) cases can lead to frustration and anger. Psychiatric patients looking for care in busy emergency rooms frequently are targets for these problems.

> The resident is called down to see a "crock" by the staff E.R. physician. The patient is calmly complaining of "seeing things." When the resident arrives, the E.R. physician is angry and comments that, "These S.O.B.'s don't belong here with people who are really sick."

How well can an evaluation be done with this kind of negative emotional response and prejudice before starting the evaluation? A request for emergency services should not be the arena for expression of personal prejudice about psychiatry or E.R. utilization by patients not deemed sufficiently emergent to the trained eye. Thus, one pitfall of emergency care is a **negative emotional response and disappointment of individual expectations** of the physician.

Emergency work is often characterized by extremes in which chaos and disruption alternate with tedium and routine (several seriously disturbed patients arriving at one time or routine sporadic evaluations throughout the day and night). This can lead to slipshod care because of situations which are too demanding, or not demanding enough. Keeping a level head, and good triage are essential in times of high demand; we can only be in one place at a time. Being alert to complexities is essential in times of low demand. Thus, a second pitfall of emergency work is the **extreme atmosphere,** which can lend itself to carelessness and disorganization.

A third pitfall is **bias about the diagnosis** before seeing the patient. In most emergency situations, the patient is frequently seen first by others (clerk, aide, nurse, etc.) before the doctor. Often, these assistants obtain a partial and inadvertently misleading history, and form conclusions which they may communicate to the physician.

> A 58-year-old, white, divorced man is seen on an emergency basis because of "alcoholic problems." On the way out of the patient's room, the aide tells the doctor, "another one for AA." The physician, after a careful interview, discovers the patient has gradually become more and more despondent after his divorce of a year ago. His alcoholic intake increased substantially at first; but now he no longer cares to eat or sleep. He feels the best thing for him may be to sell his house and leave his roots behind. Further questioned about his wish to live, he comments, "Who would miss me?" The physician decides to admit the patient. Fortunately, this doctor was able to delay his judgment until after seeing the patient and evaluating him. This enabled him to initiate the proper treatment of his depression. A less careful doctor might have brushed this off as a "routine alcoholic problem."

A final fourth pitfall is the **physician's anxiety.** Emergency work is exciting but also may be frightening. The unexpected is the rule rather than the exception. Anxiety about the uncertainty is common in anyone new to this work. Yet, when dealing with a panic-stricken, violent, or suicidal psychiatric patient, the patient needs to observe that at least the doctor is calm, which can provide the crucial psychological support to help the patient marshal his own control.

Evaluation of the Emergency Patient

In evaluating psychiatric emergencies, several principles are operative. As with all other patients, the doctor must obtain information, conduct an examination, draw conclusions and make rapid decisions about treatment. But first it is necessary to quickly establish an effective doctor–patient relationship *(rapport)*. Without this, the evaluation process will be more difficult, and far less effective.

Establishing rapport requires understanding, undivided attention, and sensitivity. One important feature of this is privacy and confidentiality. A general rule is to interview the patient before involving anyone else. The patient may request that another person accompany him. If this occurs, first request to talk with the patient alone. (Of course, if the patient is insistent, complying is better than establishing an adversary relationship.) When family members insist on accompanying the patient, politely refusing the request until after talking with the patient alone is a necessary ground rule. Because the patient may be experiencing many intrapsychic as well as interpersonal pressures, he needs an opportunity to "tell it like it is" without correction from others, or fears about their reactions. Psychiatric problems are often associated with conflict. The patient needs to know that the doctor is **his** doctor, and not everybody else's. Certainly, after an evaluation, a family session may need to take place to help clear up confusion and conflict. This is quite different from not first listening to the patient's private undistorted account of the difficulties.

The next step is to perform a psychiatric and mental status examination. Usually, this requires some modification from the standard evaluation, in that the examiner concentrates more on precipitating stressors and current situations. Emergency problems usually have a closer relationship to current events than do less acute disorders. Thus, most time is spent in eliciting the chief complaint and the history of the present difficulty. However, additional important, brief but specific, data must be obtained. This includes the past history and family history of psychiatric disorder, treatment or hospitalization; social history involving type of work, adjustment to work, quality of interpersonal relationships; and pertinent past medical history. The latter should always include

Table 1. Common Special Problems of Interviewing Emergency Patients

Problem or Complaint	Solution
1. Mute patient	Attempt to interview the patient; if unsuccessful, leave and try again later. If the patient still does not respond, interview accompanying persons. Then, do a careful physical exam and appropriate lab study and if this is negative, arrange for admission.
2. "They brought me here. There is nothing wrong with me."	Find out why "they did it to the patient." Question the patient about the nature of the relationship he has to the people who brought him. Ask why this relationship has had to progress to this point. In this way, it is possible to take the patient's side, and find out what seems to be the problem with him or someone else.
3. "Doc, I'm just nervous and don't ask me why because I don't know."	Take a careful history but don't expect the patient to be able to explain reasons for the nervousness. Ask questions about his life history in a general way and explore interpersonal relationships.
4. Patient who is incomprehensible and exhibits disorganized thought	After listening for a few minutes in an open-ended way and establishing the incomprehensibility, ask straightforward, simple, direct questions. Even though a patient is disorganized, it is possible to obtain specific history in this way.
5. Patient who appears disoriented and confused	First establish this disorientation by asking the patient if he knows where he is and what this is all about. If not, spend some time basically orienting him, and then ask specific questions about his history and current problems. If unsuccessful, proceed as with mute patients.
6. Patient who appears with extreme emotions such as fear, anger, panic, and sadness	Comment calmly, supportively, and directly on the emotional state with a statement like, "You look very frightened; tell me more about it."

asking the patient whether he is taking any drugs or medication (e.g., a patient using drugs for "recreational" purposes may answer "no" to a question about whether he is taking medications). A physical examination and review of systems needs to be done if one has not been done by a competent referring physician just prior to seeing the patient. (If there is any history suggestive of a primary or accompanying somatic problem, a physical examination and review of systems may need to be repeated, despite previous examinations.)

Although this seems quite straightforward, actual experience with patients is never quite like this. Table 1 lists some common problems

Table 1. *(continued)*

Problem or Complaint	Solution
7. Violent patient being held down by three hefty staff members with much commotion going on	Before you ask the staff to let go, have all weapons removed and say to the patient, "I would like to talk to you to find out what this commotion is all about. I need to have your agreement that you and I can talk peacefully without all these people around holding you down. If you agree, I'll ask the staff to leave." (Have the staff wait outside and be immediately available.)
8. Hostile, paranoid patient who insists there is some plot out to get him	If you are of the opposite sex to the patient, it is usually best to interview him alone. If not, requesting a staff member of the opposite sex to be present during the interview can sometimes decrease anxiety. (Paranoid patients not infrequently may be experiencing a homosexual panic.) Allow the patient sufficient space and if possible, make it clear that you are leaving an access way open for him to leave. Do not challenge paranoid delusions but begin to take the history in a general way and explore the circumstances around the onset of the suspicious feelings.
9. Belligerent, intoxicated patient	Establish from the start that you're the doctor and you wish to get more information from the patient. Assure him that no harm will come to him. Do not argue but simply state this and then listen to what he may say. It may help to have a number of staff members standing close by if he needs to be subdued. Often just a show of numbers is sufficient. If the patient is at the point of sedation, make a bed available for him to lie down. Take a history, and try to clearly establish the responsible agents. If this is not provided by the patient, obtain this history from accompanying persons. (Street drugs are often *not* what they are called, or mixtures.)

and solutions of interviewing and managing emergency patients. The problems are common but yet often can be difficult and frustrating to deal with. Nevertheless, the solutions offered can facilitate the process, assist in data collection, and clinical decision making.

The process of clinical decision making has several specific important features. Diagnostic formulation in treatment planning is an essential part of this. However, a diagnosis by itself in psychiatry as well as medicine has little practical value in caring for patients. To make a clinical decision about treatment, management and disposition, we need to be aware of six **clinical decision variables.** [This is a modification of the third edition of the *Diagnostic and Statistical Manual* (DSM III) of the American Psychiatric Association multiaxial diagnosis scheme.]

1. Psychiatric diagnosis
2. Nonpsychiatric medical disorders
3. Nature and severity of psychosocial stressors
4. Highest, lowest, and current level of adaptive functioning
5. Potential for suicide or violence
6. Availability, advisability, and practicability of possible treatment modes and disposition

The importance of the psychiatric diagnosis in clinical decision making is obvious. Seemingly less evident, nonpsychiatric complaints and disorders of psychiatric patients are no less important. Yet, they can be central or contributing factors in some psychiatric problems (e.g., "myxedema madness"), as well as being important in their own right. Psychosocial stressors are important not only in making a diagnosis (e.g., adjustment reactions) but in advising the patient about his condition. Level of adaptive functioning is particularly important because an emergency visit can be deceptive in relation to the patient's life pattern. (The chronic schizophrenic patient, despite immediate appearance, may be at a comparatively high level of adaptive function for him.) Two aspects particularly germane to emergency care are potential for suicide and violence. Finally, whatever the other concerns, one must determine if the treatment or disposition selected for the patient is an available, advisable, and practical alternative. This decision must take into account social supports, effects of removal from employment or home, etc., finances, and transportation, as well as the clinical condition.

For example, if a depressed patient who has no other disorder, has recently experienced the death of his wife, has family close by, is working, has no previous psychiatric history, has no suicidal thoughts, and has outpatient psychiatric care available, we can see how this information can lead to the decision to recommend outpatient care. Yet, if the same patient is more depressed and suicidal, lives alone, has no family nearby and no transportation, the decision about treatment will be quite different.

The rest of this chapter will discuss suicide, violence, and panic to show how these six variables can be applied to enable effective decision making.

Suicide

Suicide is generally defined as "the act or instance of intentionally killing oneself." Suicide as a clinical problem is usually a result of profound depression. Can we ever say that suicide is not the result of psychiatric disorder? This is an interesting problem for debate or research, but an irrelevant issue for the clinician. Our job is to assist anyone who is considering, planning, or has attempted suicide. One fact of note, most patients who actually commit suicide have had contact with a physician not long before. In one study (Murphy, 1977) of 60 suicides, 49 of the patients had seen a physician within the previous 6 months; 36 had given clear indications to their physicians of a primary or secondary depression. Also, more than two-thirds had a history of previously threatening or attempting suicide. Clearly, doctors must be alert to the importance of careful evaluation of suicidal possibility. How we approach this will be the subject of this section.

There are four different situations in which the problem of suicide may arise for the clinician.

1. Attempted suicide

   The patient has the intention to die, but does not succeed because of an untoward occurrence (such as an unexpected visitor who finds the patient before death occurs). A patient may also panic at the last moment and call for help.

2. Intentional self-inflicted injury or threat

   The intention is not to die but to express a feeling, manipulate others, or a plea for help. Sometimes, this is called *suicidal gesture.* It is misleading to use this term both because there may be no wish to end life, and because some of these patients accidentally succeed, or inflict grievous self-damage.

3. Reported suicidal ideation

   This patient states that he no longer wishes to live or has thoughts of killing himself, with or without active plans to do so. Any such statement must be taken seriously without question.

4. Unreported suicidal ideation

   This patient is seen because of psychiatric or medical problems such as depression, alcoholism, terminal illness or disability, schizophrenia, etc. This patient may give no direct indication of suicidal ideation, but when appropriately asked about the prospects of self-injury, he responds positively.

Evaluation of Suicidal Potential

The most important issue is **to establish the relative potential for suicide in the future.** One of the first steps is to remain unbiased about the injury or threat until you have carefully interviewed and thought through the motivation for the injury or threat. Many so-called suicide attempts may have little to do with the intention to actually kill oneself.

Table 2. Factors in the Evaluation of Suicidal Risk

Demographic Factors	Lower Risk	Increased Risk
Marital status	Married	Divorced, separated, widowed, or single
Sex	Women	Men
Age	——————Increases with age——————→	
Religion	Jews and Catholics	Protestants
Socioeconomic status	High	Low
Race	Nonwhite	White
	In the 20–25 age group, black males have a rate twice that of white men[a]	
Employment status	Employed	Unemployed
Ethnic origin	Native-born	Foreign-born

Life events	Lower Risk	Increased Risk
Giving away personal property		+
Lack of future plans		+
Living alone		+
Recent loss		+
Recent surgery and childbirth		+
No secondary gain		+
Accident proneness		+
Social disgrace—arrest, bankruptcy, disclosure of child molestation, etc.[b]		+

Yet, others which look like "gestures" may also be truly suicidal (i.e., with the intent to die). This makes the assessment of suicidal potential a harrowing experience. People injure themselves for all kinds of reasons. For example, a psychotic patient who enucleates an eye may not wish to die, but be ridding himself of the "evil eye." A young college student faced with poor grades and lack of motivation but high parental expectations may act out the conflict, and dramatically make the parents aware of this dilemma by half-hearted overdosing or wrist-cutting. Thus, he expresses anger at his parents, induces guilt in them, and may even be able to leave school. On the other hand, a markedly depressed middle-aged engineer who has lost his job and faces the prospect of a declining career may take only 20 Valiums; yet, this self-injury without seeming substance may be a true suicidal attempt unsuccessful only because of his pharmacologic naivete.

Though assessment of suicidal potential may seem to have "crystal ball" qualities, it is possible to make a reasonable judgment and advise

Table 2. *(continued)*

Clinical Factors	Lower Risk	Increased Risk
Depression		With vegetative signs, psychomotor retardation, feelings of worthlessness, hopelessness, initial phases of recovery
Severe insomnia		Even in absence of depression
Alcohol and drug abuse	————Increase with increasing use————▶	
Schizophrenia		Depressed mood, thought disorder, and suicidal ideation
Command hallucinations		+
Sexual orientation		Homosexual orientation
Physical illness	——With increased disability and pain——▶	
Family history of suicide		+
		With same-sex parent, even greater
Previous attempts		+
Lethality of attempt	Less violent and painful	More violent and painful
Hypochondriasis		+

[a]Source: Slaby, Lieb, and Tancredi, 1975.
[b]Source: Beebe, 1975.

a patient wisely about further treatment. A key factor in this judgment is establishing the intention responsible for the action. Is there a wish to die; or does motivation relate to expressing anger, soliciting help, manipulating others, etc.? The conclusion drawn may have very different implications for further management.

Evaluation of Intentionality

Four basic factors are important in assessment of intentionality:

1. Patient's explanation about the intention
2. Inferences from the severity and type of injury or attempt (lethality)
3. Inferences from statistics on risk factors
4. Inferences from the patient's historical account of his other difficulties (interpretation of unconscious motivations)

The patient's explanation is best determined by asking about it, directly and openly.

> DOCTOR: "Tell me about the circumstances which led you to hurt yourself?" (in the case of a threat—"lead you to think about hurting yourself?").
>
> PATIENT: Describes circumstances.
>
> DOCTOR: "Did you wish to die?"
>
> PATIENT: Gives answer.
>
> Toward the end of the interview—
>
> DOCTOR: "Do you still feel like hurting yourself or want to die?"

With "yes" answers to these questions, it is best to be conservative and believe the patient. On the other hand, if a patient denies any suicidal intent, we can be fairly certain that the injury or threat was not suicidal. Patients usually do not try to deceive the examiner unless there is some specific reason. (For example, a patient may fear hospitalization if he admits to suicidal intention.) One method of avoiding this is to be aware of the patient's fears by asking him about these. Once fears regarding possible outcomes of the evaluation are dealt with, the patient is unlikely to deceive the physician. If we suspect that a patient is lying or unrealistic (as in the case of delirium, dementia, or acute psychosis), we have to make a judgment of suicidal potential by inference from other data.

The more **severe and life-threatening the self-injury or attempt (lethality),** the more strongly we can infer the intent to die. In general, violent methods (firearms, hanging, jumping off buildings, etc.) indicate more serious intention.

Suicidal risk factors include a variety of demographic, clinical, and life events. The most relevant factors are included in Table 2.

Psychiatrists make **inferences about unconscious motivations** in self-injury cases. If it is determined that unconscious conflict was part of the motivation for self-injury, this judgment is made from many different perspectives (the patient's personality, type of conflict, other symptoms, etc.). But this is helpful only for those experienced in making inferences from this type of data.

To summarize, we establish suicidal potential in terms of the patient's explanation, severity and type of injury, and risk factors; and, finally, if we are skilled at interpreting the unconscious, unconscious motivations. This is portrayed in Fig. 1. We weigh these data quite carefully to make the judgment about suicide potential. For example, a single, depressed, middle-aged man living alone, who lost his only brother recently, attempted to hang himself and tells us he has no wish to live,

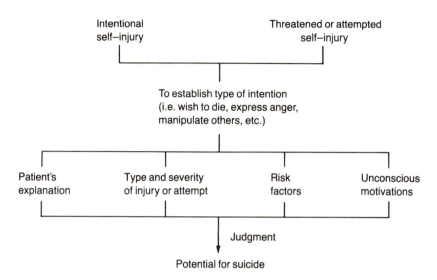

Figure 1. Evaluation of suicide potential.

would clearly be seen as intentionally wanting to die, and as a high-risk suicidal patient. A very different judgment will be made in a single, attractive, young woman, living with strict parents who tells us she has taken ten aspirins in front of her boyfriend. She tells us she did this because her boyfriend decided to break up with her; and that she hopes her parents and boyfriend realize what they have done to her.

Management and Treatment

The management and treatment of a patient with a self-inflicted injury or threatened injury involves several steps. First, a careful evaluation must be done to establish the patient's suicidal potential, as noted in the previous section. Second, a clinical decision must be made which will define the general type of treatment approach to be undertaken. This is illustrated with a case study that follows. Several other matters, however, are also important.

In cases where there has been a self-injury, the patient must be medically stabilized and able to function without extensive medical-surgical care before transferred to a psychiatric unit. Most psychiatric units are not equipped to monitor and care for patients with acute medical-surgical problems. If a suicidal patient is initially admitted and treated on a medical-surgical floor or ICU, the physicians and nursing staff in charge of the case must be alerted to the patient's suicidal potential and instructed about the degree of observations and precautions necessary (e.g., constant observation, frequent or infrequent checks). Arrangements should also be made for a psychiatric consultant to be involved in daily assessment and management.

If a decision is made that a patient need not be admitted but is referred for outpatient care, the evaluating physician must thoroughly discuss the referral with the patient as well as whoever will be responsible for providing that treatment. The patient should also be informed that if problems arise with the referral or things get worse before getting there, he should contact the evaluating physician at once by telephone to discuss the problem. The evaluating physician must be prepared to deal with the patient personally rather than merely providing the telephone number of the hospital or clinic. A "brush off" by someone unfamiliar with the case may result in progression of depressive or other symptomatology which, in turn, may lead to another suicidal episode. Establishing this *lifeline* (Beebe, 1975) can enable a simple problem to be solved by telephone without further complication. And where a mistake in judgment seems to have been made, the patient can be asked to return for reevaluation. Experience indicates that if a patient is assured that he can contact the evaluating physician directly if problems do arise, he will only do so when necessary without abusing the privilege.

Case Study

The following case history illustrates the processes of evaluation of suicidal potential and clinical decision making.

> The patient is a 56-year-old, white, married, male who was brought to the emergency room by ambulance from his hotel because of threatening to jump out of a seventh-floor window. He was stopped by the hotel manager. Apparently this occurred in the midst of a drinking bout; he had alcohol on his breath, although he did not appear intoxicated. When asked why he had tried to jump, he replied, "I have nothing to live for." He described functioning adequately until three months ago, when he sustained two successive myocardial infarctions. After recovering, he returned to work as a vocational counselor. There, he began to develop suspicious feelings about his co-workers. He felt he was slowly being pushed out of a job, despite continuing reassurance by his boss. The patient had a past history of heavy alcoholic intake approximately ten years ago. He joined Alcoholics Anonymous (AA), and was able to abstain for ten years until the last few weeks when he began drinking quite heavily again. There was no history of previous suicide attempts. After the doctor developed rapport, the patient was able to tell him that he also had long-standing marital difficulties. He and his wife slept in separate rooms. The patient had no hallucinations; nor was any further delusional material elicited. He was coherent, logical, and fully oriented. When asked if he still wanted to die, the patient indicated that he really didn't care much about that now. All he wanted was some help.

Physical examination revealed a slightly diaphoretic, overweight, middle-aged male who looked depressed and slightly tremulous. The only positive physical findings were the slight tremor of both hands, diaphoresis, and a blood pressure of 170/110.

Let us look at the six clinical decision variables (indicated on p. 144) to assist us in making the essential decisions to help this person.

1. Differential Psychiatric Diagnosis
    A. Adjustment disorder with depressed mood. Considering the absence of prior psychiatric problems other than alcoholism ten years ago, we might consider the present attempt at self-injury as a reaction to his infarction and consequent fears of job security.
    B. Major depressive episode. He feels depressed, and has some feelings of worthlessness. No history of other symptoms of depression given. With this short E.R. evaluation, this diagnosis is still a possibility and cannot be ruled out.
    C. Paranoid (or other) personality disorder. This is suggested by his suspiciousness on the job, but is an isolated finding with no prior history of suspiciousness. Some other personality disorder might be considered because of the chronic marital difficulties and excessive alcoholic intake; but to be more specific about this, we would need more data.
    D. Substance use disorder—alcohol abuse. There is a history of previous alcohol abuse with recent recurrence after abstinence for ten years.
    E. Dementia associated with alcoholism. There are no signs of intellectual or memory loss. But, in a patient with arteriosclerotic heart disease, hypertension, and an alcoholic history, there is a need for closer evaluation of intellectual functioning. Mild dementia might play a part in his functioning at work and his consequent suspiciousness.
    F. Alcohol withdrawal. Because he has been drinking for several weeks, we have to observe for symptoms of withdrawal. He already has some tremulousness and diaphoresis, which could be related to a withdrawal syndrome (or to anxiety).
2. Nonpsychiatric diagnosis
    A. Hypertension. This needs further exploration.
    B. Recent history of myocardial infarction. This and the hypertension are extremely important in further treatment decisions (e.g., prescription of psychotropic medication).
3. Nature and severity of psychosocial stressors
    Four stressors are obvious: (1) Recent myocardial infarctions; (2) difficulties with his wife; (3) difficulties at work; and (4) reestablishment of drinking. Clearly, the stress of two infarctions is severe.

The chronic marital difficulties seem to have been exacerbated since the infarctions. Perhaps his wife moved from the bedroom in fear that any sexual excitement for the patient would lead to another heart attack. Perhaps, with the patient's incapacity, his wife finally got up the strength to make a statement about chronic difficulties in their relationship. His interpretation of being pushed out of a job may or may not be accurate. Regardless of the truth, he feared that he was "over the hill," an undesirable employee. The reemergence of his old drinking pattern may be a result of other stressors, but contributes additional psychological stress as a failure experience (breaking abstinence).

4. Highest–lowest and current level of adaptive functioning

The picture seen in the E.R. is the lowest level of functioning this patient has experienced. With the exception of marital difficulties, his functioning over the past 10 years has been good.

5. Evaluation of suicide potential

He explained his attempt on the basis of "nothing to live for"; but further exploration revealed that now he just wished help. Had he actually jumped, he would likely have been killed or seriously injured (high lethality). As to risk factors, the only one which is favorable is his marital status, but even this is shaky. Finally, we can speculate about the unconscious motivations of his attempt. This could be displaced rage at his wife and his employer whom he perceives as having abandoned him, and a wish to end a life of inability and incapacity. In summary, suicidal potential is quite high.

6. Availability, advisability, and practicability of possible treatment modes and disposition

Obviously, further treatment is essential. He wants help. Diagnostic questions have not been completely resolved. Suicidal potential has been judged to be quite high.

Is in- or outpatient treatment indicated? In deciding this, we need to know some of the advantages and disadvantages of inpatient vs outpatient treatment. These are noted in Table 3.

Given his job problems, interruption of work may not be harmful, and even may be beneficial. His high potential for suicide indicates a need for a secure environment. He is at risk for an alcohol withdrawal syndrome and should have observation. Differential diagnostic questions remain; and these may require laboratory and psychometric studies. He is out of town, with no immediate supportive environment. All these factors indicate that the advantages of inpatient treatment far outweigh the disadvantages.

Thus, it is clear that methodical use of the principles outlined facilitates complete, effective clinical decision making in the suicidal patient.

Table 3. Comparison of Inpatient vs Outpatient Treatment

Outpatient Treatment	
Advantages	Disadvantages
Patient can continue functioning without major disruption	Stress is still operating
Not as stigmatizing	No immediate help available
Secondary gain features not supported	Therapy not as intensive
Maximum confidentiality	Psychometric and laboratory studies not as readily available

Inpatient Treatment	
Advantages	Disadvantages
Relatively secure environment	May be stigmatizing
24-hour nursing observation available	Expensive
Laboratory and psychometric studies readily available	Could function as rewarding secondary gain keeping him from his responsibilities
Opportunity to leave the stressful environment	Would confirm his own view of himself as incapacitated and "over the hill"
Individual and other forms of psychotherapy intensively supplied as needed	Loss of confidentiality

Violence

There is confusion about the relationship between psychiatric problems and violence. As a whole, **violence within the psychiatric patient population is exaggerated.** Violence associated with most criminal acts falls outside the purview of clinical medicine, including psychiatry. But where violence seems to have no rational aim, is associated with distortions or disorders of consciousness and thought, or involves family and intimate relationships, the involved persons are often brought for evaluation by a physician. In addition, a person may seek medical help on his own for uncontrollable rage or disorders of consciousness.

Four types of medical situations can be identified in relation to violence.

1. Active violence in a medical setting
   A patient in a hospital, clinic, office, or emergency room, who is being seen for either a medical or psychiatric problem may become violent.
2. Recent violent behavior outside the medical setting
   This patient is brought or requests an evaluation either because

of injury resulting from violence or because of a suspected psychiatric or medical disorder.

3. Reported ideation of violence

A patient may seek help for violent impulses or anger, and/or if he feels that the origin of this is some medical problem (e.g., a patient with an aura of psychomotor epilepsy who feels the urge to throw furniture). Or, a patient may be brought because he threatens violence. Finally, in the course of any medical evaluation, a patient may report an unsuspected urge to harm someone.

4. Unreported violent ideation elicited

This usually occurs when a patient is being evaluated for a psychiatric problem; and, in the course of the mental status examination, is asked if he had ever thought of hurting anyone else and responds positively.

In each of these situations, it is the physician's task to sort out the origin of violence, especially the possibility of a psychiatric disorder. Then, as with the suicidal patient, he must decide if a likely potential exists for further violence. Treatment and management decisions then are possible.

Evaluation of Potential for Violence

In evaluating violent behavior or ideation and its potential for recurrence, six factors are important:

1. Patient's complaint and explanation
2. Past history of violent behavior
3. Diagnosis
4. Childhood historical data
5. Other factors
6. Unconscious motivations

The patient's complaint and statements about plans for future violence should always be taken seriously. A patient's explanation should be listened to carefully, even if he is disturbed and irrational. For example, a psychotic may tell us that "voices" commanded him to kill a stranger because of his "suspicious" look. Until the psychosis is under control, the likelihood of injuring another person could be quite high. Yet, even a psychotic patient, in the midst of bizarre talk, may reveal that the reason he struck out at the stranger was because his wallet was being stolen.

It is important to inquire about ongoing violent ideation, for example, by a question such as, "Have you ever thought of hurting yourself or others?" As with suicide, patients rarely try consciously to deceive the physician if asked directly.

Past history of violent behavior is the best predictor of future violence. All psychiatric disorders can have violence as an accompaniment or primary component. However, two **diagnoses** stand out. These are the *psychoses* and the *impulse disorders*.

The psychotic patient, whether this is a manifestation of schizophrenia, drug intoxication, or some other organic disturbance, is characterized by a gross inability to test reality and profound disturbance in thought, feeling, and behavior. Social conventions may be abandoned. He may be hallucinating or delusional. Understanding of ordinary relationships is distorted. Sense of self may be lost. As a consequence, he may be extremely fearful and protective. Many situations which otherwise would not be threatening become a provocation (e.g., touching a patient who is behaving strangely). The stimulus may even be intrapsychic (e.g., command auditory hallucinations to kill).

Disorders of impulse control most frequently associated with the violence are the explosive disorders, and the antisocial and borderline personality disorders. The episodes of aggressiveness, while understandable, are out of proportion to precipitating events or social expectation.

A patient with an explosive disorder, which fortunately is rare, typically may describe the violent episodes as "spells" or "attacks," and, in the midst of these, may destroy property or even seriously assault a stranger. Prodromal affective or autonomic symptoms may occur. He may describe amnesia following the episode and a feeling that this behavior is out of his control. For example:

A patient is seen in the E.R. for a broken hand. The history reveals that the patient's wife told him, while they were eating dinner, that she forgot to cash his salary check. He became furious that dinner was cold and threw his plate on the floor. Angered by this, his wife left the table. The patient then put his fist through the wall, hit the frame of the house and injured his right hand. Further history revealed frequent "spells" similar to this surrounding some small failing on his wife's part.

Treatment for these disorders requires a specialist. Otherwise, and often despite this, violent episodes will continue. In episodes which involve substantial violence and family problems, it is usually necessary to admit the patient to a psychiatric unit for a brief stay until the crisis has abated. Some of these patients may be suspected of having a seizure disorder because of the prodromal symptoms and amnesia. If this is suspected, consultation from a neurologist should be obtained.

Patients with borderline and antisocial personality disorders may become violent when confronted with any type of interpersonal conflict (e.g., refusal of admission to the hospital for a minor medical problem). Treatment of borderline patients can be quite successful with expert intensive psychiatric outpatient or inpatient treatment. Those with antisocial personalities frequently do not benefit from treatment, and often go to jail. If both have been violent, the likelihood of a repeat perform-ance is high.

Childhood historical data are important to explore with questions like, e.g., "Can you tell me what life was like for you as a child?" The usual bland responses should be pursued with questions like, "I don't mean only whether it was good or bad, though that's important, but I would like you to describe what it was like for you."

Four factors are commonly found in childhood histories of violent persons: (1) parental brutality, (2) parental seduction, (3) childhood fire-setting, and (4) cruelty to animals (Beebe, 1975). The child who observes parental violence and/or is beaten unreasonably is more prone to violent methods of conflict resolution later in life. Those who experience overt (sometimes subtle) sexual seduction may later act out the guilt and frus-tration through impulsive violence or violent conflict resolution. Child-hood fire-setting and cruelty to animals are early signs of poor impulse control, as well as indicators that the child's needs were ignored. Bed-wetting, when included with fire-setting and cruelty to animals, forms a triad more frequently found in the histories of persons committing violent crimes than nonviolent crimes.

Other factors such as availability of weapons, drug, and alcohol use and abuse are also significant. In the intoxicated state [e.g., phencycli-dine (PCP) intoxication], violence is a frequent occurrence. Also, patients who come from a cultural background in which violent forms of conflict resolution are acceptable are more prone to act this way when they have a psychiatric disorder.

Although psychiatrists make inferences from **unconscious motiva-tions** about potential for violent behavior, this is rarely a useful and reliable indicator for the nonspecialist.

This is summarized in Fig. 2.

Figure 2. Evaluation of potential for violence.

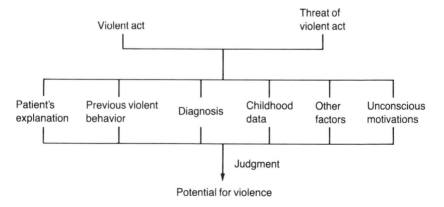

Thus, a patient who has "spells" and feels urges to be violent; who has never been violent before; who has no immediate plan or availability of weapons; who has no history of fire-setting, cruelty to animals, or bedwetting; who has no history of alcohol or drug abuse; and who is eager and willing to come back for further diagnostic evaluation to determine if these episodes are due to psychomotor seizures, may not require hospitalization. In contrast, another patient who is typically impulsive; who has been violent in the past; who is currently abusing amphetamines and now feels that if he would just stop taking drugs, all his problems would go away, may require hospitalization to assist in withdrawal and further treatment.

Management and Treatment

This is a twofold process. **First, a current violent situation must be brought under control.** Second, a clinical decision must be made about further care.

If a patient is violent in a medical setting, common sense dictates that we must stop this. A good first step is simply to calmly and firmly ask the patient to stop whatever he is doing, and talk with you. (Be certain to see that all weapons are removed before any discussion.) If this is not effective, a show of numbers, followed by discussion may be effective. If this is still not effective, it is best to call the police unless personnel trained in restraining a violent person are available. As a rule, unless the diagnosis and history are known, use of **IM or IV sedation or tranquilization is not indicated** because these interfere with neurological and psychiatric examination. For example, a delirious patient with a head injury may become a great diagnostic dilemma if sedated.

If a patient is psychotic, it is necessary to be aware that his provocation to violence may be minimal (e.g., a sudden unexplained movement toward him), and can be precipitated by poor interpersonal handling of the patient (e.g., beginning a physical examination without requesting permission; drawing blood; giving injections or fluids without warning and explanation; or not including the patient in decisions about further treatment, such as hospitalization).

Finally, **patients with impulse disorders generally are not violent in the medical setting.** However, they are often manipulative, and attempt to gain control of the physician and his decisions. They may do this by exaggerating symptoms, by complaining of psychic discomfort without any overt signs of this, or by being negativistic about recommendations other than their desired one. However, if the doctor is actively critical or indicates covertly that he does not trust the patient's reports, if he challenges the discrepancy between what is seen and reported about psychic discomfort, or if he fails to ask what the desired recommendation is before making his own, he or a staff member may be attacked. This can be avoided by realizing that these patients are very distressed, not challenging them, and negotiating a helpful treatment strategy which takes their desires into account.

The second step in management and treatment is to make a clinical decision. A case study will illustrate this process.

CASE STUDY

A 21-year-old, white, male, engineering student is brought for emergency evaluation because he beat down a dormitory door and fought with another student. He appeared fearful and anxious. The doctor introduced himself and asked if he could talk with him privately. The patient had a bag in hand containing toiletries. When asked, "What seems to be the problem," he stated "brought my bag." He was difficult to comprehend because of his extreme looseness of association. But he could respond to some direct questions. He indicated that he had not slept for three days. He denied taking drugs or medications, prior psychiatric problems, medical hospitalization, or serious illness. Asked about his childhood, he responded with a smile and no further discussion. When asked about the violence, and future plans for violence, he commented, "I couldn't understand I was leaving my body. Nobody understands. They all are not creative enough." The doctor commented on the patient's fearfulness. The patient agreed, saying he needed sleep. He then appeared to relax. The other students reported that the patient had screamed in the dormitory hall and then began pounding on the door of one of their rooms. When one of them tried to stop him, the scuffle erupted. One commented that he didn't know the patient very well because he kept to himself, but he thought that recently he was behind in his work and unable to finish an important assignment. He thought the patient might have been having some problems with his girlfriend. They reported he had not slept in two or three days. He had not been known to take drugs. Physical exam was within normal limits. Blood and urine were sent for drug screening. The patient was told quite firmly that he needed to be in the hospital to get medication and sleep. He agreed, and then was given 50 mg of chlorpromazine orally prior to going to the ward.

Analysis of the case requires an examination of the clinical decision variables.

1. Differential psychiatric diagnosis

   Brief reactive psychosis; schizophreniform disorder; schizophrenic disorder; substance-induced organic mental disorder. A *brief reactive psychosis* involves acute psychotic symptoms appearing after an identifiable psychosocial stressor, with no prior period of increasing psychopathology. Some of the stresses experienced by this student (work and girlfriend problems) would not ordinarily be seen as extreme enough to precipitate this severe a reaction by themselves. However, sleep deprivation in combination with these could have been involved.

The patient fits the picture well enough for it to be the best working diagnosis. The diagnosis of *schizophreniform disorder* would be considered in this case if the duration of illness turned out to be longer than several weeks. If further family history reveals evidence of schizophrenia, and later follow-up reveals he has persisting residual symptoms, the diagnosis of *schizophrenic disorder* may be correct. The diagnosis of *substance-induced disorder* is possible, but unlikely because of the negative history and any physical signs of drug effects (pupillary changes, tremor, hyperpyrexia, etc.).

2. Nonpsychiatric diagnoses
   None discernable.

3. Nature and severity of psychosocial stressors
   The two stressors in this patient's life do not appear to be of the severity to warrant such an extreme reaction. However, sleep deprivation may have tipped the balance.

4. Highest, lowest, and current level of adaptive functioning
   This was the low point in the patient's lifelong functioning by available history.

5. Potential for violence
   This is a rather typical case of violence associated with psychosis. The patient was not purposefully, intentionally wishing to harm anyone, but also was unintentionally provoked into a violent confrontation by others attempting to stop him from hurting himself or destroying property.

   In summary, we clearly have an irrational patient who will not rationally answer questions about violence, has been violent recently, is clearly psychotic, and gives no childhood or drug history. Without the proper treatment, the immediate future potential for violence is high.

6. Availability, advisability, and practicability of possible treatment modes and disposition
   This patient is most likely in the midst of a brief reactive psychosis. He is away from home in a relatively nonsupportive environment. His potential for further violence is high. Consequently, the advantages for inpatient care far outweigh the disadvantages. He should be hospitalized on a psychiatric unit.

Panic

Panic may be defined as a feeling of "sudden overpowering terror." It can be a manifestation of a discrete primary panic disorder, which is characterized by frequent panic attacks occurring at unpredictable intervals, and which requires referral for intensive psychiatric treatment. Or, it can be secondary to some other psychiatric or medical disorder. The terror of panics may be presented verbally by a patient as **somatic complaints:** "My heart is beating too fast. It is going to stop. I'm having a heart attack. I can't breathe, I'm going to suffocate. I'm going to die." **Physical signs** of panic may include such things as tachycardia, agitation, hyperactivity, diaphoresis, tremor, and hyperventilation. **Psychological complaints** may include such statements as, "I think I may be going crazy; I'm losing my mind; I must be having a nervous breakdown; I'm so confused." In all of these expressions, there is one common characteristic, frightful anticipation of extreme impending doom.

Panics can be secondary to a generalized anxiety disorder or neurosis, drug intoxication and withdrawal states (particularly amphetamine, cocaine intoxication, and LSD "bad trips"), or to acute schizophrenia and delirium. **Physical disorders** such as hypoglycemia, pheochromocytoma, and hyperthyroidism can be accompanied by panic, or the patient may have similar but less severe symptoms. Occasionally, patients with major depressions and somatization disorders may develop panics. A particular type of phobia, agoraphobia (fear of being alone or in public places), with panic attacks precipitated by the attendant feelings of helplessness or being overwhelmed, is an important differential diagnosis since treatment with tricyclics may relieve the panic attacks. Phobic

Figure 3. Differential diagnosis of panic.

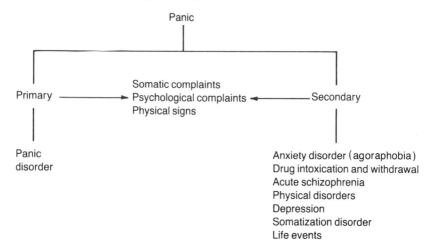

patients may become panic stricken when exposed to the fearful stimulus. Panic may also be elicited by sudden unexpected life events such as the accidental death of a loved one, loss of a job, natural disaster such as a fire, or following a violent attack such as rape or mugging. Figure 3 summarizes the differential diagnosis of panic.

Management and Treatment

The management and treatment of panic involves **careful evaluation to determine if the panic is a primary disorder** or is accompanying one of the other conditions noted above. If the panic is not a result of a primary disorder, we must treat the underlying problem. (For example, if the panic results from amphetamine intoxication, we will need to hospitalize the patient, use neuroleptics, and be prepared to handle the depressive "crash" following withdrawal.) Following careful evaluation, **short-term treatment of acute panic has features which are similar regardless of whether the panic is due to a panic disorder or is secondary.** These features are control of the situation, identification of the object of fear if possible, and medication.

First, **the physician must be under evident control of himself as well as the situation.** A patient in panic can terrify others and communicate his fright to all involved. An interactional spiraling process can occur, increasing the patient's panic. It is helpful to separate the patient and accompanying persons if they are very upset. (But many such patients feel secure only with familiar persons; so that this may be impossible. Then, it may be wise to start with the others present and to gradually separate them.)

Second, the patient may be so preoccupied with his immediate state that his awareness of its origins is absent. Despite this, a careful history may reveal the **object (stimulus) of the fear.** Common objects of fear are fear of incurable disease (death) or insanity, homosexuality, abandonment, inadequate sexual performance, occupational failure, and revenge for past misbehavior. If the doctor can identify this with the patient, that process may alleviate much of the acute picture. In addition, future panic responses may be eliminated if a recommendation can be made for appropriate follow-up care (e.g., marital counseling for an extremely dependent person panicked by an impending marital separation).

Finally, in someone who will not respond to an empathic and orderly approach, administration of an **anxiolytic agent or neuroleptic** may be appropriate depending on the underlying condition. (Benzodiazepines are usually used for this purpose and should be given orally or IV because of poor IM absorption.) The patient may then be able to talk to the physician, and gain reasonable control over this overwhelming feeling.

CASE STUDY

A 57-year-old, single, female sales clerk is seen as a walk-in emergency. She is in an extremely agitated state; she complains of her heart beating "too fast." Her anxiety had been increasing over the past few months, and escalated a few weeks ago, upon the death of her sister. She had been treated in the past by her physician with very large doses of oral diazepam as her somatic preoccupations increased. Recently, he discontinued this because it did not seem to help. She described a 40-year history of multiple varied somatic complaints, for which all previous workups were negative. As the discussion progressed from her somatic concerns to the sister's death, she began to regain control of herself. She was given a prescription for diazepam, told the dosage would be gradually tapered over the next few weeks and given a follow-up appointment for the next week. Analysis of the case can now turn to review of the clinical decision variables.

1. Psychiatric diagnosis

     This patient presents a picture typical of chronic somatization disorder with longstanding mild anxiety. The latter escalated into a panic reaction after sudden discontinuation of a high level of antianxiety medication and the recent death of her sister. She responded to empathic discussion with the physician. Her object of fear, i.e., having an incurable disease and dying (like her sister) was not identified by her previous physician.

2. No nonpsychiatric disorder

3. Psychosocial stressors

     As outlined above in item 1, "Psychiatric diagnosis."

4. Adaptive functioning

     This patient's usual way of adapting to stress was to use somatization. This was not sufficiently adaptive in this situation. She rapidly decompensated but just as quickly responded, returning to her previous level of functioning.

5. Potential for suicide or violence

     There was no history of violence or suicidal ideation.

6. Availability, etc.

     Since she responded in the office to the current approach, further outpatient treatment was available, practical, and agreed to.

Conclusion

Psychiatric emergency states are commonly seen in all areas of medical practice. Their differential diagnosis, management, and treatment can be greatly facilitated by a systematic approach. There is no substitute or shortcut for careful evaluation and thoughtful clinical decision making. Better patient care and fewer complications are the rewards.

Additional Readings

Beebe JE: Evaluation of the suicidal patient. Evaluation and treatment of the homicidal patient, in Psychiatric Treatment Crisis/Clinic/Consultation. Edited by Rosenbaum CP, Beebe JE. New York, McGraw-Hill, 1975, Chapters 2 and 4

Diagnostic and Statistical Manual of Mental Disorders, 3rd ed. (DSM III). Washington, DC, American Psychiatric Association, 1980

Gerson S, Bassuk E: Psychiatric emergencies: An overview. Am J Psychiatry 137:1–11, 1980

Lazare A, Eisenthal S, Wasserman NL: The customer approach to patienthood. Arch Gen Psychiatry 32:553–558, 1975 (This is an informative and interesting article describing the interpretation, elicitation, and negotiation of patient requests.)

Murphy GE: Suicide and attempted suicide. Hosp Pract 12:73–81, 1977

Skodol AE, Karasu TB: Emergency psychiatry and the assaultive patient. Am J Psychiatry 135:202–205, 1978

Slaby AE, Lieb J, Tancredi LR: Handbook of Psychiatric Emergencies. New York, Medical Examination Publishing, 1975

PART V

PSYCHOSOMATIC MEDICINE

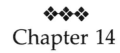

Chapter 14

Psychosomatic Medicine
The Psychosomatic Approach;
Psychosomatic Disorders;
Psychiatric Disorders with Somatic Symptomatology

Donald Oken

One sometimes hears a patient or a condition referred to as "psychosomatic." To use the term this way perpetuates a basic misconception. There are no "psychosomatic disorders" nor "psychosomatic patients" because there are no **non**psychosomatic disorders or patients. Psychosocial factors enter into every state of illness, as they do in the healthy state of all people. **All disorders of all patients are psychosomatic.** To divide diseases into "organic" or "functional" is misleading, despite its seeming commonsense utility. Both elements are involved in all disorders, including those in the traditional province of psychiatry.

Other similar "commonsense" medical dichotomies are equally false. Who has not had experience with a young, single woman whose period is delayed after a sexual exposure? How is that to be defined? Is she sick or well? Normal or abnormal? Is her condition organic or functional? Is her anxiety cause or effect of the delay? Is her visit to her physician diagnostic or therapeutic? The supposed separate poles of all these dichotomies actually overlap. Each is correctly defined in more-or-less terms for each patient, depending on the specific factors characterizing that patient: psychological **and** biological **and** social. And they shift over time. The physician's job is to elicit information about all these factors and to incorporate this in an overall (bio-psycho-social) treatment program. This is the only correct clinical usage of psychosomatic medicine.

This applies to every patient. When a diabetic comes to the physician out of control, there is more to the job than administering insulin, correcting the acidosis and electrolyte imbalance, and adjusting diet. Complete diagnosis includes understanding the reasons for the dyscontrol;

and treatment must be directed to these. Psychological stress itself is capable of precipitating acidosis. Rebellious defiance may motivate refusal to take insulin, a common occurrence in diabetic children. Depression may result in inattention to both insulin and diet. Even when infection or trauma are the main culprits, the doctor must learn how and why these occurred. Was there self-destructiveness or poor judgment related to the exposure? Was hypoglycemic confusion induced by overzealous self-treatment involved? Perhaps psychological stress contributed to low resistance, as is known to occur. The diagnosis of diabetic acidosis is merely the initial, incomplete step in understanding the patient.

Another dimension is *illness behavior*, the degree to which a patient considers himself "sick" and decides whether to see a doctor. Delay, with pauses enroute for self-medication or "consultations" with family, friends, or druggists can play a role in the development of the disorder. Another patient may rush to the doctor at the first sign of minor discomfort. These attitudes also help determine how seriously the doctor's "orders" will be taken.

It has been reported often that about half the patients who consult physicians have "no organic disease." While incorrect as stated, what this truly means is that half our patients suffer from an illness in which psychological and social factors are more prominent or immediately relevant than biological factors. Many have disorders which pose no life threat, and most often are chronic. Politely, they are often called psychosomatic patients. Less so, they are termed "crocks." Either way, the notion is that they are sick in some different way—or not sick at all. As a consequence, they are poorly treated. Those doctors who avoid these terms because they appreciate the essential nature of all illness as psychosomatic, in contrast, can provide very effective treatment by applying that knowledge, whether or not the patient has some major "disease."

"Psychosomatic Disorders"

Disorders in which there is demonstrable organ pathology, in which psychological (and social) factors are believed to play a primary etiological role have sometimes been referred to as "the psychosomatic diseases." The list of these, which varies among authors, most commonly includes peptic ulcer, essential hypertension, rheumatoid arthritis, bronchial asthma, ulcerative colitis, and thyrotoxicosis.

The assertion that the psychosomatic mechanism in these disorders is distinctive and etiologically more significant than in other disorders remains doubtful. Suggestive evidence comes from the finding that the patients with each condition tend to exhibit specific psychological characteristics, either in their overt personality or deeper makeup (psychodynamics). But most people with these characteristics never develop the given disease. And analogous patterns are seen in other disorders not in this group—probably excluded because biological causal factors were identified earlier. (One such example is the "Type A" behavior pattern associated with coronary artery disease, characterized by time urgency, job involvement, and a hostile, driving competitiveness.) The presence of these patterns seems incontrovertible, although their key features require further elucidation. But it is entirely possible that the psychological and biological features are **both** products of another primary biological defect, for example, a genetic predisposition.

The demonstrated high correlation between stressful life events and the appearance of the disease or its attacks also has been placed in evidence. But, as already indicated, this is true for all illness, which is one basis for understanding every disorder as psychosomatic. We cannot conclude that this relationship is stronger for this particular group of disorders.

Without doubt, psychological factors play a significant role in the disorders called psychosomatic. Perhaps, historically, some purpose was served in using that term to underline that this is true for disorders with incontrovertible "organic" pathological lesions, as it is for "functional" disorders. But this is no basis for separating the two.

Substantial research since the 1950s has clarified the presence and nature of psychosomatic mechanisms in a variety of normal and clinical states. But none of it has established that the mechanisms in this "psychosomatic" group differ from those in all other disorders. Possibly, later studies will reveal quantitative or other differences. Even if so, almost certainly these will be of epidemiologic significance rather than relevant to treating a given patient. Conversely, even if a breakthrough reveals undisclosed biological etiological factors for any of these disorders, this will be added knowledge which in no way erases the validity of existing relationships with personality or life events.

Some authors have used the term *somatopsychic* as a classification for patients in whom psychological symptoms, including disproportionate disability, arise as an apparent reaction to the presence of a disease and its symptoms. Use of this separate category is equally unwarranted. The same is true of the parallel term *psychological overlay*. Every patient has a psychological over- and underlay which represents aspects of the picture of his illness. It is merely that for some patients these factors are more **maladaptive.** If so, it is the correction of these dysfunctional features, more than the biological dysfunctions, that treatment must address primarily.

The basic **therapeutic approach** to "psychosomatic," "somatopsychic," and all other patients is the same. This centers on use of the doctor–patient relationship to obtain the type of history that includes data on life events and their meaning to the particular patient. It matters not whether the disease is life-threatening or less grave. When a disorder is chronic, there is opportunity to nurture the relationship and to provide, within its growing strength, supportive medical psychotherapy. For these patients who develop awareness of their psychological problems, or in whom these are of sufficient extent to warrant the additional diagnosis of a psychiatric disorder, referral for psychotherapy is indicated. It is best to emphasize the psychological benefits of such a procedure, rather than imply that it will have specific somatic benefits, though these may well occur.

Psychiatric Disorders Presenting with Somatic Symptomatology

Certainly, all psychiatric disorders have somatic features. They too are psychosomatic. From a practical standpoint, behavioral disturbances ordinarily predominate, so that their somatic components present no special problems. But it is well to keep in mind also that the presence of any one disorder is no insurance against developing another. Every complaint and physical sign must be an object of serious diagnostic scrutiny.

Somatic symptoms are a major feature of some psychiatric disorders, however. This situation presents problems of diagnostic differentiation. This is a common occurrence in medical practice. Patients consult their regular physicians for help even when they suspect the basis is psychiatric. The stigma, guilt, and fear associated with psychiatric illness and psychiatrists augments this. It also enhances the tendency to focus initially on respectable somatic complaints as a legitimate "admission ticket" to get the doctor's help. Because the patient fears that the doctor may share these prejudices, and disapprove of him, behavioral and psychosocial problems often do not emerge until the patient safely observes that the doctor does not react negatively to him or to preliminary hints of the true nature of the problem.

Anxiety Disorders

The symptoms of these typically include sympathetic hyperactivity, with its usual symptoms. At times, only one of these may be sufficiently prominent to motivate complaint, e.g., palpitation. But careful history will reveal others, as well as subjective anxiety. Actually anxiety disorders are less common than often thought. The term *anxiety state,* or *chronic anxiety,* often is misapplied as a generic term for any or all psychiatric disorders producing somatic symptoms.

Depressive Disorders

These present several problems. Somatic symptoms such as sleeplessness, constipation, dry mouth, and sexual dysfunction are common presenting complaints. The frequent combination of anorexia, weight loss, and lack of energy suggests malignant disease. The patient may **not** experience or complain of being sad, but only of loss of interest or energy, especially the geriatric patient.

Paranoid Disorders

These patients may present with somatic delusions, the underlying persecutory quality of which may require exploration to elicit. ("What do you think may be causing your 'belly pains'?" . . ."Electric currents" . . ."Electric currents?" . . ."Yes, they have my house wired to find out if I tell what I know.")

Malingering

This diagnosis rests on determining the sought-for advantage which being ill is consciously expected to provide (secondary gain). Usually this soon becomes evident. Narcotic addiction may be involved. The symptoms may suggest any disorder, medical or surgical, but usually don't quite fit, being patterned on the lay concept of the disorder, rather than its actual clinical features.

Factitious Disorders

These are more difficult to detect. They involve the actual production of a pathological sign (e.g., placing blood in the urine) or a lesion (e.g., via excoriation). These patients can be very clever in mimicking other disorders, especially because a disproportionate number are health personnel. The activity itself is quite conscious. But conscious advantage is absent or minimal. Rather, the motivation is unconscious primary gain involving very deep-seated trends of masochism, exhibitionism, hostility, and dependency. Referral to a psychiatrist expert in psychotherapy is mandatory. Unfortunately, many refuse and depart angrily. The key factor here—as in malingering—is that referral be made in a sympathetic, nonjudgmental way. These patients are very ill, if not in the way they suggest. If this is done, even a patient who leaves in a huff may return later to get help. Diagnosis often requires hospitalization, with exquisitely careful control of circumstances around tests or specimen collections (e.g., having a nurse present while obtaining the temperature). But resort to ruses to trick the patient are counterproductive, and too often used. "Grilling" a patient also is inappropriate. In whatever way the diagnosis is revealed, it is never appropriate to view it in the context of discovering dishonesty, or to confront the patient with the inconsistency "caught." The doctor is neither police officer nor judge, but a helper.

Accident Proneness

A more subtle problem, this diagnosis should be considered in anyone who suffers repeated trauma, even as a pedestrian. The typical patient is young, somewhat impulsive, usually male, and inclined towards risk taking in leisure activities as well as everyday life. The problems are deep-seated and unconscious, though not necessarily grave. They can be resolved only in intensive psychotherapy. A less common variant is the patient whose accidents arise from the poor judgment and planning, and often poor coordination, arising from an undetected organic mental disorder.

Conversion Hysteria

These patients can develop any of a variety of somatic symptoms (e.g., pain, seizures) or dysfunctions (e.g., paralysis). Typically the patient talks freely about the symptoms in gory detail, while being vague on other historical facts. Despite the dramatic, exaggerated quality of the words, he seems remarkably calm: *la belle indifférence*. In this country, hysteria is most common in females, the young, uneducated, and unsophisticated. "Epidemics" may occur in groups, mimicking food poisoning or an obscure infectious disease. Classically, the symptom pattern fits the lay pattern of disease but not the physiology (e.g., "glove anaesthesia"). But symptoms can correspond closely to other disorders (e.g., coronary pain or renal colic) because they are modeled on relatives or friends who had these, or on a prior illness of the patient. There may be secondary gain. Episodes of hysterical illness tend to be transient and readily responsive to warm supportive care and a **brief** period of indulgence. But they may be recurrent, involving the same or other symptoms. Inappropriate surgery must be avoided. If recurrences develop or episodes fail to clear quickly, psychiatric referral is essential. With chronicity, prognosis worsens sharply.

Somatization Disorder (Briquet's Syndrome)

This is likely a variant of chronic hysteria of a more malignant type, though perhaps unrelated. **These patients are often labeled "crocks" or "hypochondriacs."** But, unlike those patients sometimes also called crocks or "psychosomatic" merely because psychosocial factors are especially relevant in their illnesses, this group has major psychopathology. They have multiple symptoms in multiple-organ systems. Not uncommonly, they report several episodes of unsuccessful (in retrospect, inappropriate) surgery. They make a career of illness, with innumerable visits to doctors and hospitals. The neurological, female reproductive, gastrointestinal, and cardiopulmonary systems are involved with great frequency, though symptoms may be difficult even to classify. Pains are common. Complaints tend to have a hysterical quality of dramatic exaggeration combined with vagueness; and often are shifting and recurrent. Sexual inhibitions and dysfunctions are common. Some patients do moderately well, with few restrictions in life functions other than those due to the time spent in medical care. Others are severely or totally disabled. This disorder is far more common in females, but may be underdiagnosed in males. Careful history will reveal its onset to be in the teens or early 20s. The prognosis is often very poor and treatment exceedingly difficult.

Underlying psychopathology is severe, with evidence of covert depression, dependency, and masochism, not always easily discerned by the nonpsychiatrist. And they are inapparent to the patient except as justifiable reactions to somatic discomfort. Thus, these patients rarely accept or benefit from psychotherapy. The disorder has become an entrenched way of life, associated with multiple, subtle, secondary gains which complicate the basic psychopathology. Illness behavior has become life behavior. The physician can only regard these as patients with a chronic incurable illness.

Treatment centers on support, interest, and **limited** symptomatic therapy. Medication side effects fit right into the psychopathology, becoming magnified, and complicating diagnosis as well as subsequent treatment. Drugs of abuse or addiction are avoided, for problems with these are frequent. Consultations should be kept to a minimum, though often urged by the patient. Surgery is fraught with the near-certainty of subsequent complications ("adhesions"), and should be used only for unequivocal indications. Gentle but firm refusals to requests for inappropriate medication and surgery are essential, but may result in doctor-shopping. The latter is minimized if the doctor indicates his concern for the patient and for the real, if psychogenic, suffering. Treatment works better if the doctor indicates that it may be helpful rather than curative, and that the patient is bearing up bravely in the face of a terribly uncomfortable, but not dangerous condition. Assurances that a treatment will work typically result in a return visit during which there is an almost triumphant report of its failure.

Hypochondriasis

Most patients incorrectly called hypochondriacs fit into the previous disorder. Technically, this term is reserved for a very different and **rare disorder.** This involves massive preoccupation with bodily functions, usually with the fixed belief—often amounting to a delusion—that a dread somatic disease is present, such as cancer. It may be related to the major depressive or paranoid disorders; and features of one or the other sometimes can be elicited. After thorough medical workup, including those tests indicated by the complaint, the physician must indicate with absolute firmness that there is no evidence the feared disorder is present, and that the real problem is the worry about it. The physician can readily combine this stance with an acknowledgement of his lack of omniscience and stated willingness to follow the patient. Attempts to convince or argue with the patient are fruitless. The fear is irrational and not amenable to logic. No amount of unindicated tests, x-rays, etc., will assuage the patient's concern, though he will urge these. Their use simply prolongs the situation and adds cost. Psychiatric referral should be recommended; usually is refused; but may eventually be accepted. Or his family may pressure him to go. Antidepressant or neuroleptic medication may help, but are best left to the psychiatrist in this difficult situation. Psychiatric hospitalization may be required.

In all these disorders, diagnosis rests both on positive and negative features. A complete standard medical workup is always indicated, and the various nonpsychiatric disorders ruled out. But diagnosis cannot be made by exclusion alone. Positive evidence of the psychiatric disorder must be sought for. In their genuine absence (not merely the failure to uncover or recognize them) the diagnosis must be deferred for further studies.

Anorexia Nervosa: A Paradigm of the Psychosomatic Problem

Anorexia nervosa illustrates aptly the oversimplification involved in separating off and categorizing diseases as psychosomatic, psychiatric, or organic. This serious condition involves gross disturbances in both psychological and somatic functions. Much more common in females, it typically first appears in the later teens or early 20s. The problem centers on a decrease in eating. But its name is misleading because actual loss of appetite is rare initially, though common later. Periodic episodes of binge eating are common, sometimes dramatic in their grossness. Induced vomiting is common. Excessive activity (exercise, athletics, etc.) is frequent, both for its own sake and as a weight-loss device. There is intense concern about eating, and body size and conformation. The emphasis these patients place on weight loss is extreme. They use all sorts of ruses to continue the process and to keep others unaware of its extent so as to prevent interference. Patients vary through the full range of severity, as may different episodes in the same patient. Some literally starve themselves to death. Amenorrhea is almost invariable in females.

Major changes occur in body protein, in the composition and distribution of the body fluids, and in endocrine functions, which require careful attention. Overt psychopathology is ubiquitous, but varies greatly in extent. The largest group have a borderline personality disorder, a condition notoriously difficult for the nonpsychiatrist to diagnose. Some seem to be hysterical. A few are psychotic. Characteristic severe disturbances in body image are present that can be confirmed by testing. A peculiar complex of intrafamily pathology has been noted in many patients, requiring psychotherapy of the entire family. **Treatment** is never easy. Combined treatment by pediatricians (or internists) and psychiatrists with special expertise in this disorder is preferable; and essential in more severe cases. Hospitalization for a time may be necessary, even life-saving.

Additional Readings

Drossman DA: The problem patient. Ann Int Med 88:366–372, 1978

Engel GL: Psychological Development in Health and Disease. Philadelphia, Saunders, 1962

Engel GL: The need for a new model: A challenge for biomedicine. Science 196:129–136, 1977

Grinker RR: Psychosomatic Research. New York, Norton, 1953

Lipsett DR: Medical and psychological characteristics of "crocks." Psychiatr Med 1:15–25, 1970

Oken D: Psychosomatic theories, in International Encyclopedia of Neurology, Psychiatry, Psychoanalysis, and Psychology. Edited by Wolman BB. Cincinnatti, Van Nostrand-Reinhold, 1977

Strain JJ: Psychological Interventions in Medical Practice. New York, Appleton-Century-Crofts, 1978

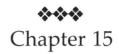

Chapter 15

Chronic Pain

Anthony E. Blumetti

Without doubt, the most common symptom which patients present to a physician is pain. To the extent that the patient can describe the pain, its distribution and its precipitants, diagnosis can be facilitated. Pain complaints vary considerably, not only from patient to patient but also from one medical setting to another. The acute pain symptoms presented by some patients in emergency settings, often indicative of serious pathology, may be different from those symptoms presented by a well-known, recurrent patient in an ambulatory setting. All pain complaints should be thoroughly investigated. It is important to distinguish immediately between benign pain, not indicative of dangerous pathology, and malignant pain which indicates more critical or terminal illness. Complete medical workup, including laboratory and x-ray evaluations, aid in this differentiation.

Not uncommonly, there are patients whose pain persists over a long period of time (over 6 months) despite a variety of treatment modalities, even though no specific, clear-cut organic etiology is directly related to the quality or intensity of the discomfort. Even when somatic pathology is present, it seems insufficient to explain the extent of the pain and disability. The pain complaints take on a major focus in their lives. It is just these patients who prove the most difficult cases to handle in practice. They are often diagnosed as having a "psychogenic" component to their illness, or "psychosomatic" difficulties. They can be characterized as suffering from states of tension, stress, depression, frustration or suppressed rage; and may have a history of psychological difficulties, poor interpersonal relationships, poor family life, etc. A related variant is the patient who is disposed to polysurgery and/or polydrug use, and who cudgels the physician into prescribing more medication or referral for more surgery. If the physician feels that he is being manipulated into this position against his better judgment, a reevaluation of the case is in order. When patients are on heavy doses of narcotic medication without relief, drug dependence or abuse problems must be considered.

It is important to define and differentiate four terms often misused in describing these patients: (1) conversion hysteria; (2) psychophysiologic reaction; (3) hypochondriasis; and (4) somatization. A *conversion disorder (conversion hysteria)* refers to an alteration or loss of physical functioning with no organic disorder in which the symptom is an expression in symbolic form of some psychological conflict. Histrionic personality traits such as lability of affect, repressive defenses, overconventionality, etc., are usually present. Examples of conversion disorder include paralysis, dyskinesia, and anesthesia. This diagnosis is never used unless other evidence of hysteria accompanies the pain.

A *psychophysiologic reaction*, also referred to as a psychosomatic condition, is present when psychological factors affect a physical condition of known organic etiology. Often depression is present, as a reaction to a long-standing physical problem, which then in turn contributes to the condition. Tension headache, angina, cardiospasm, neurodermatitis, and sacroiliac pain are examples of these.

Hypochondriasis is a preoccupation with the belief of having a serious illness or disease, approaching (or reaching) delusional proportions. Immense energy is invested in physical signs, sensations or changes, which are interpreted as abnormal or evidence of serious illness. Secondary gain and manipulation are often present.

Somatization occurs when there are repetitive, multiple physical complaints of several years' duration for which medical attention is frequently sought. These patients often have a complicated medical history with somatic complaints in multiple systems, described in dramatic, exaggerated terms. Anxiety and depression may also occur. Patients who use somatization have very few resources to fall back on to deal effectively with the world; and hence resort to focusing on their bodies in an infantile way to exert some control on the world and get attention.

Unfortunately **most chronic pain patients do not fall neatly into any of the above four diagnostic categories,** but usually present with characteristics which are multidescriptive. The diagnostic category of *psychogenic pain disorder* has recently been established (in the third edition of the *Diagnostic and Statistical Manual* [DSM III] of the American Psychiatric Association) for these patients. This refers to a clinical picture where the predominant feature is pain in the absence of explanatory physical findings **and** evidence of psychological factors.

There are also a sizable number of patients with chronic pain where psychological factors arise only secondarily to long-standing discomfort from definite organic pathology. Examples of these are patients with rheumatoid arthritis, musculoskeletal difficulties due to postoperative scarring and adhesions, temporomandibular joint syndrome, etc. Anger, frustration, anxiety, and depression can result, causing disruption of vocational, social, and interpersonal functioning, as well as interfering with an ongoing treatment process.

No matter what the classification of the pain syndrome, **one paramount task is to make some determination on the basis of the clinical interview (see Chapter 1) as to whether a psychogenic component to the pain symptomatology is present.** Keeping in mind the characteristics of patients falling into the aforementioned diagnostic categories, certain cues should be focused upon in a structured interview to aid in decision making. These cues fall basically into nine categories, as follows:

1. Overinvolvement in invalid status
2. Control of life by pain
3. Involvement of significant others in symptomatology
4. Dependence behavior
5. Satisfaction with life
6. Avoidance behavior
7. Subjective experience of pain
8. Financial gain
9. Degree of emotional involvement

Overinvolvement in invalid status refers to how invested an individual is in being sick. Listening to how patients describe their symptoms is most important. Overinvolved patients describe their pain in extreme emotional terms, i.e., "terrible," "excruciating," "intolerable," etc. Doctors and treatment procedures are described in exacting and minute detail in terms of time, place, and person. The patient sees his symptoms as making him an invalid, and seems to attain gratification from this.

When considering **the amount of control pain has had** over the patient's life, one must inquire into work, recreational, interpersonal, and sexual pursuits. The criterion here is whether there has been cessation of activities in these areas or continued functioning.

When **involvement of family members or significant others in symptoms** takes place, some type of secondary gain (e.g., sympathy, attention) is usually present. One must ascertain the degree to which family life and activities center on the patient and his limitations, and whether the patient relies inappropriately on others most of the time for help or assistance.

Closely related to this is **dependence behavior,** and the patient's ability and desire to take an active role in his treatment program rather than being passive and letting doctors "cure" him. Excessive use of medication and/or alcohol to deal with problems is also an important indication of excessive dependency.

It is not unusual for chronic pain patients to **find their lives unsatisfying,** and to have been unfulfilled in job, marriage, and social relationships even before these symptoms began. One should also learn whether any major life events occurred just prior to the beginning of symptoms, such as death of a spouse, divorce, change of job, financial problems, etc. The degree to which a patient sees extraordinary demands placed on him over which he has no control also adds to the possibility of a psychogenic component. When these perceived demands become overwhelming, pain can function to allow **avoidance** of demands or expectations, not only at work but also in home and family life, social relationships or sexual functioning.

A useful method of obtaining the patient's **subjective experience** of pain is to observe his discomfort through his behavior during the interview (shifting around in bed or chair, grimacing, holding body rigidly, etc.). He is then asked to rate his level of discomfort on a scale of 0 to 100, where 0 is no pain and 100 the most severe pain experienced. Extreme discrepancies between the clinician's and the patient's estimates in either direction may point to a psychological component of the pain symptoms.

Financial gain for pain should always be considered, particularly because many chronic pain conditions are due to work related injuries. Patients often receive workmen's compensation, disability income, etc. If someone earns relatively more being disabled than working, there is little incentive to recover. The clinician must not be timid in asking details of the present financial status. Also pending litigation is a very strong incentive for the patient to keep his symptoms, since he may fear he will not be compensated adequately for his discomfort and missed work if he improves significantly.

Finally, the degree of **emotional disturbance or involvement** must always be evaluated. This is particularly true of depressive mood, hostility, anxiety, lability of affect, and somatic fears or delusions. This judgment can be made aside from a formal mental status examination. Often sufficient information will be obtained by the interaction with the patient and self-reports of his symptoms or problems.

In general, when a patient is under any type of stress or in the throes of psychological turmoil perceived to be out of his control, a feeling of helplessness takes over, and habitual coping mechanisms begin to break down. Any sensory input can be seized upon and exaggerated to help explain the misery. Thus, pain threshold can be lowered; and pain can act as an escape or mediating device between the patient and his interaction with the world. In this way, pain often carries a message when its subjective report appears out of proportion to the presumed or diagnosed condition.

When a significant psychological component to the patient's pain problem is suspected, referral for formal **psychological testing** can be advantageous to confirm the clinical impression, and to determine the extent and nature of the psychological difficulty. The Minnesota Multiphasic Personality Inventory (MMPI) has been the most widely used instrument in the evaluation of pain patients. The profile obtained is compared to profiles characteristic of various clinical groups. For chronic-pain patients, the amount of hypochondriasis, hysterical defenses, degree of affective involvement, oral dependent character traits, etc., can be ascertained. Other tests, such as the Rorschach inkblot test, may be used to determine underlying psychological conflicts, impairment of ego defenses, level of psychosexual development, and ability to gain from various forms of psychotherapy.

Treatment of the chronic pain patient is a very complex endeavor, which can be not only frustrating, but also an emotionally taxing experience, not uncommonly leading to pain management rather than treatment. Supportive counseling and a trial on medication can be helpful. If it becomes apparent, however, that the psychological problems are complex or well entrenched, referral must be made to a psychiatrist or psychologist experienced in handling chronic-pain patients, or to a specialized pain clinic.

If analgesics are used, the choice is dictated by the origin, quality, intensity, and duration of pain. Medication can be characterized as non-addictive (aspirin, phenylbutazone, etc.); moderately addictive (codeine); and strongly addictive (morphine and its derivatives) agents. A trial on tricyclic antidepressants in combination with analgesic medication may prove useful, especially for the variety of patients whose psychological symptoms are limited primarily to agitation and depression. In most cases, this should be done in consultation with a psychiatrist. If the physician finds himself in the position of utilizing strongly addictive agents and is becoming involved in prolonged pain management or maintenance of his patient, referral is a must.

Various noninvasive treatment methods such as psychotherapy, biofeedback, relaxation, and stress-reducing techniques, etc. have been used in pain management and treatment. These are best handled by experts in the field. Since not all patients are responsive to these interventions, a careful evaluation must be done by the psychiatrist or psychologist to whom the patient is referred. If a special pain treatment service is available, this most likely utilizes a multidisciplinary approach, with an emphasis on behavioral management of pain including control of medication, dealing with family problems, enhancing stress-reducing skills as well as an active physical therapy and vocational counseling program. It will usually be expected that the referring physician maintain contact with the patient and the pain specialists, not only for better follow-up but also to avoid the patient's feeling "dumped" or pushed out, which may add to his distress and help perpetuate the pain.

Additional Readings

The Behavioral Management of Anxiety, Depression and Pain. Edited by Davidson PO. New York, Brunner-Mazel, 1976

Diagnostic and Statistical Manual of Mental Disorders, 3rd ed. (DSM III). Washington, DC, American Psychiatric Association, 1980

Melzack R, Chapman CR: Psychologic aspects of pain. Postgrad Med 53(6):69–75, 1973

Pinsky JD: Aspects of the psychology of pain, in Chronic Pain. Edited by Aue BL. New York, Spectrum Publications, 1979

Chapter 16

Sleep Disorders

Joyce D. Kales and Anthony Kales

Normal Sleep

There are two major types of sleep. *Rapid eye movement (REM) sleep* is associated with most normal dreaming experience and has characteristic electroencephalograph (EEG) patterns. *Non rapid eye movement (NREM) sleep* is composed of sleep stages 1, 2, 3, and 4, which represent progressively deeper sleep levels as defined by auditory thresholds necessary for awakening. The typical night of sleep for the young adult begins with a short period of stages 1 and 2 sleep followed by a longer period of stages 3 and 4 sleep. After approximately 70 to 100 minutes of NREM sleep, the first REM period occurs. From this REM period, the sleeping individual reenters stages 2, 3, and 4, swings back through stages 3 and 2, and ultimately returns to REM sleep. This cycle is then repeated at approximately 90-minute intervals throughout the night. Most of stages 3 and 4 sleep occurs in the first half of the night, while REM and stage 2 sleep predominate in the second half of the night.

The proportion of REM sleep is highest in the newborn, and decreases in early childhood to stabilize at 20 to 25% of total sleep time through adult life. The amount of stages 3 and 4 sleep, which is highest in childhood, progressively decreases, so that in the elderly these stages are minimally present or totally absent.

Insomnia

Insomnia is the sleep disorder most frequently encountered by physicians. Over 40% of the adult population report having had difficulty sleeping at some time in their lives. Insomnia can take the form of difficulty falling asleep, difficulty staying asleep, early final awakening, or combinations of these. Sleep laboratory studies have shown that although the clinical complaint of insomnia is usually valid, insomniacs tend to overestimate the severity of their sleep difficulty, sometimes greatly.

Insomnia is a symptom not a diagnosis. It can be caused by psychological factors, situational circumstances, medical conditions, or pharmacologic agents. A complete history (and examination) is essential for diagnosis. This includes special attention to a general sleep history, psychiatric history, and drug history. The general sleep history includes the type of insomnia, the nature of its onset, and the duration, severity, and frequency of sleep difficulties. It is important to obtain a 24-hour, 7-day history, as well as evaluate environmental factors and the general family and work situations.

Situational insomnia is most often transient and related to **life stress** events such as difficulties with work or family, or personal loss.

Pain, physical discomfort, and distress due to **physical illness** are obvious enemies of sleep. When the discomfort is mild or unfamiliar (e.g., minimal orthopnea) the patient may be unaware of the primary disorder and complain only of insomnia.

Various **pharmacologic agents** also can interfere with sleep directly; and **"rebound insomnia"** following withdrawal of hypnotic drugs is common. The drug history includes evaluation of the patient's consumption of coffee, cola-type drinks, or alcohol, as well as previous pharmacologic treatment for insomnia. Overtreatment is frequently a problem with hypnotic drugs since the ineffectiveness of most of these drugs may cause the patient to increase the dosage, leading to hypnotic drug dependence.

Sleep disturbance is extremely common in patients with **psychiatric disorders.** It is a typically prominent feature of depressive illness, and may be the presenting symptom. **Particular attention should be directed to eliciting signs and symptoms of depression** in otherwise unexplained insomnia. Insomnia is frequent in other major psychiatric disorders, including schizophrenia, mania, and organic mental disorders. Not uncommonly, it represents a significant issue for patients with chronic psychoneurotic illness or personality disorders, whose complaints may be the most persistent and difficult to manage. A complete psychiatric history can usually point out a relationship between the onset of chronic sleep difficulties and psychological conflicts or major life stress events.

Treatment should include the encouragement of patients to gradually increase their daily activity and exercise, to regulate their daily schedules, and to go to bed only when they feel sleepy. When insomnia is mild, these measures may be sufficient in themselves, while in severe insomnia they can be useful adjuncts to psychotherapy and pharmacologic treatment.

Generally, the treatment of insomnia associated with depression or other major psychiatric disorders is best accomplished as part of the primary treatment of the disorder itself. Moreover, the drugs used for these have, in most cases, intrinsic hypnotic properties. The physician can capitalize upon this for dealing with the insomnia by judicious selection of the particular agents in these drug classes which have maximal sedating properties (e.g., chlorpromazine or thioridazine; amytriptyline or imipramine[1]), and by giving most or all the required dose at bedtime. Undertreatment with the tricyclic antidepressants may be a problem, however, if the sedative effects are confused with the basic actions of these drugs, with insufficient attention to residual insomnia. If necessary, flurazepam (15 to 30 mg) can be added at bedtime. Usually this can be discontinued once the primary treatment becomes fully effective.

When insomnia is associated with a transient disorder, (e.g., life stress, acute physical or psychological illness, or brief exacerbation of chronic illness) short-term treatment with a hypnotic may be indicated,[1] along with treatment directed to the primary cause. **Flurazepam is the drug of choice.** Treatment is usually initiated with 15 mg at bedtime, which may be increased to 30 mg. **Barbiturates should be avoided.**

When hypnotic drugs are indicated as adjunctive treatment for chronic insomnia, flurazepam is cautiously recommended. Flurazepam is a long-acting benzodiazepine hypnotic whose effectiveness with continued use (up to 1 month) has been demonstrated in many laboratory and clinical studies. The long-acting metabolites contribute to a carry-over effectiveness during the first few nights following withdrawal, and may facilitate either a temporary or total withdrawal from the drug. In addition, unlike the withdrawal of shorter-acting benzodiazepines, withdrawal of flurazepam has not been shown to be accompanied by rebound insomnia. However, patients taking long-acting benzodiazepines should be warned about decrements in daytime performance that may accompany persistently high blood levels of active drug and metabolites. Also, many authorities believe that no hypnotic should be taken for longer than 1 month. Thus, the potential advantages and disadvantages of long-acting benzodiazepine drugs such as flurazepam need to be thoroughly considered and balanced in the total treatment of the patient.

Disorders of Excessive Sleep

Narcolepsy

This relatively rare condition is characterized by **recurrent attacks of daytime drowsiness and irresistible sleep, usually associated with one or more auxiliary symptoms** of this disorder. These auxiliary symptoms

[1]See also Chapter 21, Psychopharmacology.

include (1) *cataplexy*—episodes of partial or complete loss of muscle tone usually induced by strong emotions or sudden stimuli; (2) *sleep paralysis*—a temporary loss of muscle tone and resulting inability to move that develops in the state between arousal and sleep; and (3) *hypnagogic hallucinations*—vivid auditory or visual perceptions that occur during the transition between wakefulness and sleep, particularly while falling asleep. The peak age of onset of narcolepsy is between 15 and 25 years of age.

The diagnosis of narcolepsy is confirmed by the presence of cataplexy and other auxiliary symptoms. About three-fourths of all narcoleptics have cataplexy. If sleep attacks are the only symptom, all-night sleep and daytime nap diagnostic EEG recordings may confirm the diagnosis by detecting a sleep-onset REM period, since narcoleptics characteristically begin their sleep with a period of REM sleep rather than NREM sleep, which is typical of normal sleepers.

Misconceptions that the narcoleptic patient is lazy, dull, malingering, or suffering from an underlying psychiatric disturbance commonly result in secondary psychological disturbances. To prevent this, the family and employer should be counseled on the nature of the disorder. The patient should also be cautioned not to drive, to operate machinery, or to perform other critical tasks when he is not functioning optimally.

In **treating the sleep attacks,** methylphenidate is the drug of choice. To avoid the development of tolerance, the physician should prescribe the lowest possible dose on a p.r.n. basis, and encourage daytime naps and drug holidays whenever feasible.

Hypersomnia

This condition is characterized by periods of excessive daytime sleepiness and sleep that usually are longer than narcoleptic attacks. Nocturnal sleep is generally prolonged, but otherwise may not be disturbed. It usually begins later in life, often between 30 to 40 years of age. In idiopathic hypersomnia, there is often a positive family history for hypersomnia or narcolepsy, and sleep drunkenness (difficulty in fully awakening in the morning) is frequently a symptom. Psychogenic hypersomnia is usually secondary to a depressive disorder; not infrequently, hypersomnia is the presenting symptom of neurotic depression.

If one has eliminated psychogenic hypersomnia as the diagnosis, analeptic or stimulant drugs, preferably methylphenidate, are indicated to treat the excessive diurnal sleepiness, prolonged nocturnal sleep, and sleep drunkenness of idiopathic hypersomnia. When medication is indicated for psychogenic hypersomnia, in addition to psychotherapy, a **non**sedating tricyclic antidepressant such as protriptyline should be chosen.

Sleep Apnea

Sleep apnea, which often is a life-threatening disorder, has been reported most frequently in patients with disorders of excessive sleepiness (narcolepsy and hypersomnia), and rarely in patients with a primary complaint of insomnia. In patients with hypersomnia associated with sleep apnea, there is excessive daytime sleepiness and sleep attacks (often indistinguisable from narcoleptic sleep attacks) associated with respiratory abnormalities during sleep. The incidence of sleep apnea is not known, but it is far more frequent in men than women.

There are three types of sleep apnea: central, peripheral, and mixed. *Central apnea* is characterized by the simultaneous interruption of both oral and thoracic breathing, and their simultaneous resumption. In *peripheral (obstructive) apnea*, thoracic respiratory movements persist after the interruption of oral respiration. *Mixed apnea* is characterized by the initial cessation and subsequent resumption of thoracic movements concomitant with interrupted oral breathing.

In evaluating any patient for sleep apnea, it is important to question the spouse, parent, or other family member for the presence of interrupted nocturnal breathing associated with snoring, gasping, gurgling, choking, periodic loud snorting, or morning headache. The snoring patterns associated with sleep apnea are characteristically unique: there are 10- to 40-second periods of suspended respiration followed by very loud and abrupt snorting sounds of about 2 to 4 seconds' duration.

In patients with obstructive sleep apnea who are obese, weight reduction may be helpful. Many patients with obstructive apnea may require a tracheostomy, however. Imipramine (Tofranil) may be helpful in treating patients with central apnea.

Sleepwalking and Night Terrors (Pavor Nocturnus)[2]

Sleepwalking and night terrors are more common in children than in adults. Sleep laboratory studies have shown that these disorders tend to occur early in the night out of deep (stages 3 and 4) NREM sleep. During a sleepwalking episode, the individual appears to be **confused, detached, and relatively unresponsive**. Night terrors are more dramatic; patients manifest intense terror and panic, and there is extreme autonomic discharge and vocalization. In both disorders, patients are difficult to arouse, and complete amnesia or minimal recall of the episode is frequent.

Both sleepwalking and night terror patients often have positive family histories for either or both disorders, and the two disorders sometimes

[2]See Chapter 11, Common Behavioral Disorders of Childhood, for further discussion of these topics.

occur in the same patient. Both disorders typically begin in childhood or early adolescence, and are usually outgrown by the end of adolescence, suggesting a delay of CNS maturation. **Significant psychopathology may be suggested, however, when one or more of the following factors is present: late onset** (after about age 12); **frequent episodes** persisting more than several years; **lack of a family history** for sleepwalking or night terrors; or **disturbed daytime behavior.** These factors indicate a need for psychiatric referral.

The **primary concern in managing patients** with sleeping or night terrors **is to protect them from injury.** Special safety measures should include latches for outside doors and bedroom windows, ground floor sleeping accomodations, and removal of dangerous objects. Episodes should not be interrupted if such an intervention previously has added to the confusion and fright of the patient. Parents should be reassured that in most cases the child is not psychologically disturbed and will outgrow the condition. Psychological disturbance is more frequent in adults with these disorders and often warrants psyciatric referral. Benzodiazepine drugs that suppress stage 4 sleep, such as diazepam, have been reported to control night terrors and may be used in adults as adjunctive treatment. We do not, however, recommend the use of these psychotropic drugs in children.

Nightmares[3]

Nightmares, in contrast, **occur during REM sleep.** They may occur at any time of the night, but are much more common later in the sleep period when there is a greater proportion of REM sleep. **Patients usually awaken spontaneously, reporting vivid and detailed dream recall,** and often have trouble returning to sleep.

Nightmares in children are usually transient and situational. When nightmares persist in either children or adults, other symptoms of psychopathology are usually present. In these cases, psychiatric referral should be made. Physicians first should rule out the possibility that frequent nightmares **may be related to the use or withdrawal of CNS-acting drugs** which result in alterations in sleep and dream patterns.

Enuresis[3]

Enuresis, or bed-wetting, occurs in over 10% of all children older than age 4. In primary enuresis, the child has never had a consistently dry period lasting more than 1 month; in secondary enuresis, the child may

[3]See Chapter 11, Common Behavioral Disorders of Childhood, for further discussion on these topics.

be dry for several months or years before a relapse in bed-wetting occurs. Children with primary enuresis often have a positive family history for the disorder, and usually have a small functional bladder capacity. In secondary enuresis, psychological factors are often causative, reflecting regression or a need for attention.

Evaluation includes obtaining a thorough history, physical examination, and urinalysis. The physician determines if the enuresis is primary or secondary, and if secondary, the time of onset and the surrounding circumstances. On physical examination, the physician notes the child's general growth and development, assesses the urine stream, determines the urine's specific gravity to assess the concentrating power of the kidney, and evaluates functional bladder capacity.

Parents of children with primary enuresis should be counseled that parental mishandling of the situation can create guilt and anxiety in the child and may result in psychological problems. Bladder training exercises are often recommended for children with primary enuresis. In cases of secondary enuresis, psychiatric referral should be made after organic causes are excluded.

Additional Readings

Guilleminault C, Tilkian A, Dement WC: The sleep apnea syndromes. Ann Rev Med 27:436–484, 1976

Kales A, Caldwell AB, Preston TA, Healey S, Kales JD: Personality patterns in insomnia. Arch Gen Psychiatry 33:1128–1134, 1976

Kales A, Soldatos CR, Caldwell AB, Kales JD, Humphrey FJ, Charney DS: Somnambulism: Clinical characteristics and personality patterns. Arch Gen Psychiatry 37:1406–1410, 1980

Kales JD, Kales A, Soldatos CR, Caldwell AB, Charney DS, Martin ED: Night terrors: Clinical characteristics and personality patterns. Arch Gen Psychiatry 37:1413–1417, 1980

Soldatos CR, Kales A, Kales JD: Management of insomnia. Ann Rev Med 30:301–312, 1979

Zarcone V: Narcolepsy. New Engl J Med 288:1156–1165, 1973

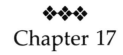

Chapter 17

Sexual Problems in Medical Practice

Eugene A. Kaplan

Sexual problems are among the most distressing human problems for which patients consult physicians. Such concerns are very personal and difficult to share with another person. For these reasons, when a patient finally feels sufficiently comfortable to bring up sexual problems or concerns, sympathetic and thoughtful listening to what the patient has to say is crucial. In addition, the physician must understand the various types of sexual problems and their causes, and be willing to advise in those areas in which he is competent, or to refer appropriately when his time or skill is limited. Physicians in the primary care areas see the vast majority of patients who present with sexual problems, and can handle a number of the more common, less psychologically complex difficulties themselves.

The Sexual History

Taking a sexual history requires skill, knowledge, and tact. A **full** sexual history is rarely indicated in the course of the general medical history. However, **within the framework of a general medical history, a physician should give every patient an opportunity to bring up any questions or concerns about sexuality.** Such open-ended questions as, "Are there any sexual problems or concerns you would like to discuss," are usually sufficiently unstructured and nonthreatening so that those patients who do wish or need to bring up such problems will have an invitation to do so, while those who do not will not feel that the physician has been unduly prying.

When the patient does mention a sexual problem, a more extensive sexual history is in order. This inquiry is least threatening if the physician initially focuses questions on the particular topic that the patient has brought up, and keeps initial inquiries unstructured, giving the patient an opportunity to describe his problem in his own way and in his own words. More detailed questions can then follow, to help set this problem in the context of the patient's general sexual history and experience, and medical and psychosocial background. Areas which seem particularly stressful or troubling should be approached with especial tact, and noted by the physician who must decide whether these are personally troubling to the patient, or more a reflection of general antipathy toward certain sexual experiences or practices. Most patients will be more comfortable giving information about current sexual activities and then relating earlier experience, practices, and concerns.

Sexual Problems in the Male

Problems can arise in any of the three phases of the sexual cycle: desire, arousal, and orgasm. The most common problems in the male include premature ejaculation, retarded ejaculation, impotence, and sexual disinterest.

Premature Ejaculation

This is **primarily, although not exclusively, a young man's problem.** A patient is considered to be a premature ejaculator if he routinely ejaculates prior to vaginal entry, immediately after entry, or so quickly after starting intercourse that either he and/or his sexual partner usually fail to fully enjoy the sexual act. (Although some authorities have suggested a timing criterion, e.g., ejaculation within 30 seconds of entry, a functional definition makes far better sense.)

In general, premature ejaculation comes about because of **anxiety about intercourse coupled with a very excitable or "trigger happy" sexual reflex** in the younger male. Most adolescent or young adult males are naturally capable of a very rapid sexual cycle from the moment of first arousal and erection to the moment of ejaculation. If this capacity for rapid sexual response, itself neurophysiologically normal for this age, is accompanied by undue anxiety about intercourse, an individual may ejaculate prematurely. If substantial anxiety about intercourse, including performance fears, impregnation fears, or even fear of venereal disease, becomes a major force in the patient's sexual life, a **habit** of ejaculating prematurely may well become established. This in itself creates still more anxiety about the next sexual act, making another episode of premature ejaculation even more likely. Some patients, of course,

have additional, deeper anxieties about their own sexuality or participation in sexual activity; these, too, can contribute or be major factors.

The most useful **treatment program** for the majority of these patients
has been Masters and Johnson's (1970) modification of Seman's technique of squeezing the glans of the penis shortly before the male feels
he is about to ejaculate. This usually works best when both the patient
and his sexual partner are counseled and participate in the treatment
program. Essentially, this involves a slowing down of the sexual reflex
through a momentary mild aversive technique just before the male
reaches the point of ejaculatory inevitability. It is essentially a recondi-
tioning or relearning procedure, in which the male is taught to maintain
his erection but to delay the ejaculatory response. For most younger
men with premature ejaculation, this treatment, plus **the context of
reassurance** in which it is offered, is sufficient to successfully treat the
problem. For a smaller number of patients with deep-seated anxieties
or aversions to intercourse, more complex counseling or psychotherapy
is necessary; and such patients should be referred for this type of therapy.

Delayed Ejaculation

Ejaculatio retarda is a **much less common** ejaculatory problem. It is
characterized by an inability to ejaculate for a very long period of time
despite full erection and substantial genital stimulation. This problem
usually arises in those men who, for one reason or another, have unconsciously come to see ejaculation as a dirty, soiling activity, and consequently inhibit their ejaculatory response automatically, even though
they are able to maintain an erection and participate in intercourse.
Often they come from strict religious or cultural backgrounds in which
there was a strong inhibiting sanction against genital sexuality, which
was then unconsciously translated into an inhibited ejaculatory response. Some patients also have difficulty trusting their partners, a feeling which also can contribute to the problem. Patients with ejaculatio
retarda do not usually respond to brief interventions and **generally require more extensive therapy** or counseling about their sexual inhibition.
For these reasons, such patients are not usually treated by primary care
physicians but rather are best referred to specialists in this area.

Impotence

Impotence, an arousal phase disorder, is the inability to initiate or to
maintain an erection sufficient for intercourse (or other sexual activities).
It is the **most common sexual problem for the older male,** in contrast
with premature ejaculation.

There are **physical, i.e., organic causes** which may require investigation, including diabetes, multiple sclerosis and other neurological conditions, vascular disorders, debilitating diseases, drug or alcohol abuse, testosterone deficiency, prolactin excess, hyperthyroidism, and certain common medications. Among the latter are antihypertensives, major tranquilizers, narcotics, antiandrogens, etc. When organic causes are suspected, a more detailed medical history and physical examination are indicated. Serum testosterone determinations may help in identifying testosterone deficiency; and a more elaborate endocrine workup of the hypothalamic–pituitary–gonadal axis may be indicated when other common causes or organic impotence are ruled out.

A good history can help differentiate psychological from organically caused impotence. If a patient has the capacity to have erections during sleep or on arising, and/or the capacity to have erections and ejaculate through masturbation, the biological equipment is likely to be working properly. In ambiguous cases, a urologist can arrange a nocturnal penile tumescence test. While the majority of impotence is psychogenic, the possibility of organic causes should always be considered and appropriate treatment instituted, if indicated.

Impotence is generally divided into two classes: primary and secondary.

Primary Impotence is the failure to **ever** have the experience of full erection and ejaculation. It is a rare condition which requires a full medical (including endocrine) workup. Usually it is due to **deep psychological problems** which can only be treated with extensive psychotherapy.

Secondary Impotence is defined as the **loss of the previous ability** to become sexually aroused, have an erection, and complete the sexual act. It usually comes about because of life stresses or traumatic events, or problems involving either the individual himself or his relationship with his sexual partner. Common stresses include physical illness (e.g., recent heart attack), personal failure or loss, depression, marital discord or problems with the sexual partner, major financial reverses, fears of venereal disease, fatigue, and fears of aging, death, or dying. External toxins such as drugs and alcohol can also inhibit or undermine the sexual response. Once a man has had an experience of being unable to get an erection and maintain it, he is likely to become increasingly anxious about what will happen next time. If this recurs, it further reinforces his anxiety and inhibits subsequent attempts at intercourse. A cycle of sexual failure followed by anxiety about the next "performance," followed by more failure becomes established.

The treatment for this condition depends very much upon the cause. If the secondary impotence has come about because of a simple and potentially reversible situational stress, then the treatment involves relieving that stress. If, however, the problems go deeper or are related to longer-term conflicts between the sexual partners, then therapy must be directed at these underlying causes. The conjoint sexual therapy developed by Masters and Johnson (1970), and the sexual therapy technique devised by Helen Singer Kaplan (1974) are both useful in reestablishing a better sexual relationship in those couples where the relationship itself has become the source of the difficulty. These amount to a kind of reeducation of the couple. Both partners are taught to relearn to experience bodily pleasure (through "sensate focus" and "pleasuring" exercises) while the pressure for successful sexual performance is removed. They also learn to communicate with each other more openly and resolve interpersonal difficulties contributing to the male's erectile problems. (One couple who referred to their experience with Masters and Johnson as a "second honeymoon" were coming closer to the truth than perhaps they realized, given one of the functions of the first honeymoon.) In this context, impotence is understood as an expression of difficulty between a couple which can best be treated by working with both partners, rather than as simply a problem of the individual.

Sexual Disinterest (Inhibited Sexual Desire)

Some men lose interest and enthusiasm for sex over a number of years, far above and beyond the mild decrease which accompanies normal aging. This loss of desire can come about for either psychological or biological reasons, sometimes both. Common psychological issues include boredom, fatigue, loss of interest in the sexual partner, unconscious anger toward the partner, loss of physical attractiveness, anxiety about decreasing performance and aging, or experiences of rejection at the hands of the sexual partner. Physical causes can include androgen deficiency, overuse of drugs or alcohol, diabetes, cardiovascular problems, urological or neurological difficulties, and many others. Often the problem is brought to the attention of the physician not by the patient himself but by his sexual partner. The patient is often reluctant to discuss this, either out of embarrassment, or because he is content with the status quo and does not want the physician to interfere.

If the patient does decide or agree to define this as a problem that he wants to do something about, there are ways to help regenerate or revive this flagging sexual interest. If the patient is older, a thorough medical history and physical examination are warranted, as well as a sexual history directed toward the current problem. Again, as with secondary impotence, simple life stresses and situational problems can be addressed by the primary physician. If the problems are deeper and/or involve major difficulties in the relationship with the sexual partner, as is frequently the case, these should be referred to appropriate therapists.

Sexual Problems in the Female

As with the male, problems can arise in any of the three phases of the sexual cycle: desire, arousal, or orgasm. The most common problems in women are sexual unresponsiveness, orgasmic unresponsiveness, and vaginismus.

Vaginismus

This relatively **uncommon condition** is characterized by an involuntary tightening or spasm of the muscles guarding the entry to the vagina such that penetration is difficult or impossible. This is usually profoundly distressing to both the patient herself and to her sexual partner. **Most women who have developed vaginismus have done so because of a prior history of major sexual or genital trauma.** The spasm or "locking of the gate" is an involuntary and automatic response to the fear of repeated trauma, even though the woman consciously may not see sexual activity as traumatic. Some patients who have vaginismus will give a history of forced entry or rape, or in some cases medical violation of the body with inadequate preparation during childhood or early adolescence.

Treating this condition frequently requires a two-level approach involving the combined efforts of a knowledgeable, sympathetic gynecologist or urologist as well as a sexual therapist. First, remembering and thorough empathic discussion of the original traumatic incident(s), if such existed, is often very helpful. Second, a conditioning approach is tried, in which the woman is helped to gradually accept the gentle exploration and penetration of her vagina, first by her own fingers or a graduated series of vaginal dilators which she, herself, controls. Proceeding at a relaxed pace, the introduction of her own hand, subsequently her sexual partner's hand and eventually the penis, can be accomplished, if done gently.

Orgasmic Unresponsiveness

Large numbers of women enjoy sex but do not necessarily know how to experience orgasm. Woman's capacity for orgasm seems to be less automatic than is the male's, although whether this is culturally or psychobiologically determined is still a matter of conjecture. Many of these women can be helped to become orgasmic, if they would so like. Some of the psychological issues that retard or inhibit orgasm in women are analogous to those which in men produce impotence and other sexual problems. For the woman, these frequently include fears of "letting go";

anxiety or guilt about sexual behavior, including masturbation; conflicting notions about the woman's appropriate role and activity in a sexual encounter; and negative or ambivalent feelings about the specific sexual partner. Such concerns, anxieties, and cultural programming may well inhibit the sexual response, especially orgasm. **Counseling with skilled sexual counselors or therapists** has been helpful to many women when the problems are relatively simple. Most anorgasmic women can learn to achieve orgasm by self-stimulation; and subsequently many can learn also to achieve orgasm in response to clitoral stimulation by a sexual partner. A somewhat smaller group may learn to extend this to full intercourse. Sexual counseling is useful in helping a woman develop these capacities, as well as work out underlying sexual or interpersonal problems, when present.

General Sexual Unresponsiveness (Inhibited Sexual Desire)

Even more commonly than the male, the female can be sexually unresponsive generally. This lack of desire can be due to psychological or physiological factors, or their combination. Psychological factors include a loss of interest in or affection for the sexual partner (partner rejection); anger toward the partner; depression; a paradoxical fear of success or intimacy; a belief that sexuality is inappropriate, bad, or dirty; a loss of self-esteem; early cultural or familial conditioning about the meaning of sexuality; a reawakening of childhood sexual inhibitions; and/or a turning of attention toward children, a career, or other interests rather than sexual activity. In addition to the usual biological factors, such female-specific biological factors as nursing, with its hormonal concomitants, or menopause may contribute to a desire-phase disorder.

As with male impotence, sexual disinterest can either be primary or can occur in women who previously enjoyed sexual experiences but, for some of the reasons listed above, are "turned off." Here, too, **treatment** is best directed toward the underlying cause. If the issues are simple and there has been a recent precipitating stress or situation which has brought about a cessation in sexual interest, then giving a woman an opportunity to deal with or work through that problem via brief therapy may help restore her to her usual sexual function. This approach is often coupled with a series of experiential tasks (Masters and Johnson's "pleasuring") in which both the woman and her partner participate together. The function of these tasks is to gently reintroduce the woman to pleasureful bodily experiences, decrease inhibitions, and experience sexual pleasure in a safe and comfortable setting. However, if problems are more deep-seated and long-lasting, it is necessary, if the patient is willing, to explore these with a qualified psychotherapist.

Additional Readings

Green R: Human Sexuality: A Health Practitioner's Text, 2nd ed. Baltimore, Williams & Willkins, 1979

Kaplan HS: The New Sex Therapy. New York, Brunner-Mazel, 1974

Kaplan HS: Disorders of Sexual Desire. New York, Simon & Schuster, 1979

Kinsey AC, Pomeroy WB, Martin CE: Sexual Behavior in the Human Male. Philadelphia, Saunders, 1948

Kinsey AC, Pomeroy WB, Martin CE, Gebhard PH: Sexual Behavior in the Human Female. Philadelphia, Saunders, 1953

Masters W, Johnson V: Human Sexual Response. Boston, Little, Brown, 1966

Masters W, Johnson V: Human Sexual Inadequacy. Boston, Little, Brown, 1970

Simons R, Pardes H: Understanding Human Behavior in Health and Illness. Baltimore, Williams & Wilkins, 1977, Chapters 21–25, pp 220–282

Chapter 18

Difficult and Obnoxious Patients

Donald Oken

The ideal physician who never has an unkind feeling about a patient is, like a dragon, a mythical beast, and an undesirable one. Only robots lack feelings. Negative feelings arise from the same human capacity that allows us empathy and compassion. Some patients we like better; some less well. These variations reflect our personality, values, and background, and the way each of these mesh with such characteristics of the patient. At times, even our favorite patients annoy us. Within wide limits, the negative feelings we develop are inconsequential to our therapeutic effectiveness.

A few patients stimulate stronger feelings that do interfere. A number of these simply represent one of those odd mismatches between a particular pair of personalities. Usually, they soon depart to another doctor, to the benefit of all. But others have a proclivity for distressing their doctors that is more general and serious.

Before considering these, it is essential to understand that our negative feelings, unpleasant and antitherapeutic though they can be, also can be useful. **The doctor's emotional reactions to a patient provide invaluable diagnostic information.** They are major indicators of the motivations and adaptive style of the patient. They suggest how the patient relates to others, who are very likely to be affected similarly. They serve also as initial clues for recognizing certain typical groups of difficult patients, which, if confirmed, can be used to develop an effective therapeutic approach.

Psychiatrists are specially trained to recognize subtle experiences of their feelings arising in diagnosis and therapy. These are particularly useful in identifying traits associated with personality disorders. The felt sense of being drained, for example, suggests a patient's dependency. Such emotional reactions represent prototypical "reflex" responses to the behavior of others. Nasty behavior begets anger, revealing the patient's nastiness; sexual arousal suggests seductiveness; and so forth.

There are important caveats, however. The doctor must be sure that the source of his reaction is the patient, not something in his own life (including a prior patient). The pattern must be pervasive, not just responsive to a specific event. Also, the doctor must precisely identify the characteristic of the patient serving as a stimulus from among the alternatives. The patient who engenders exasperation may do so because he is so confusing, not nasty; and this may be due to schizophrenic thought disorganization, organic impairment, manic tangentiality, etc. Finally, **this in no way suggests that the doctor express his feelings to the patient,** though ventilation to a trusted colleague may help.

Many psychiatric symptoms upset or revolt the average person, a prime factor in the widespread lay prejudice against the mentally ill. The well-trained, responsible physician has little of this response. What part he does develop is used to help make the diagnosis and to proceed with appropriate medical and psychiatric treatment.

But there are certain patients whose behavior is so blatantly disturbing that they can drive us up a wall. Their behavior is not only offensive, it interferes with efforts to provide essential medical care. This flies straight in the face of what we are most committed to do. Hence these patients stimulate feelings of dread, despair, fury, and hate. The intensity of these feelings is such that their recognition is rarely a problem. But they do stimulate shame and guilt; and if these become too intense, we may do ourselves the disservice of hiding our reactions from ourselves. If, instead, we accept them as normal reactions, we can use their presence as indicators that we are dealing with someone who fits into one of a group of disorders aptly called difficult, obnoxious, or hateful patients. That knowledge arms us with ways of dealing with them which make them more amenable to treatment. Thus, our negative feelings lose their sting, and become easier to bear.

The Self-Willed, Counter-dependent Patient

These are among the easiest of this group to "take." They have many traditional virtues, admired and often shared by doctors. They are successful achievers, embrace responsibility, complain little, and are dependable and decisive. In routine care, they present few problems, though they are likely to be impatient with the restrictions of treatment and poorly compliant. When they become seriously ill, the significance of these problems become evident. They thwart efforts at restriction and treatment as if they were not ill, and go one better by behaving in an opposite fashion. Our admiration rapidly becomes admixed with intense frustration and anxiety.

This reckless denial of illness reveals the real situation. Their personality traits represent an extreme, if ordinarily effective, denial of opposite tendencies, of which they are ashamed: needs to be cared for and helpless fears that the doctor will fail to meet these needs.

One patient, who suffered a coronary, illustrates the problem and its management. In the face of orders, he insisted upon walking to the lavatory, and shaving, grooming, and exercising daily. Insisted is the wrong term, he simply did this. He also conducted his business uninterruptedly via telephone, becoming heatedly involved in decision making. Attempts to get him to desist by explaining the dangers were not only fruitless, they provoked outbursts of anger and refusals to take medication, which justly alarmed the staff even more. Only when the behavior was understood could effective treatment begin. His coronary diagnosis was reexplained more casually, with emphasis on his strength and vigor in physiologically adapting to his heart damage, rather than its dangerous potential. A bedside commode was installed. He was convinced to design a plan for temporary reorganization of his office with delegation of his responsibilities. Then, his executive skill was enlisted in several real administrative problems within the hospital, the solution to which required only thoughtful paperwork. With all this, his truculence disappeared; and he cooperated with treatment.

In essence, **treatment of these patients focuses on allowing them to keep their fears hidden and to maintain their counter-dependent adaptive pattern, in ways that interfere least with treatment.** As in the example, compromises are required. But these put far less strain on the compromised myocardium than the earlier behavior.

The Clinging–Dependent Patient

At the other pole, are those patients who never get enough of the doctor. The problem is not so much their primary illness, which may be serious (or not), but their illness behavior. They go on at length about their symptoms, problems, and concerns, for which they require lengthy explanations, reassurance, advice, and symptomatic treatment. Getting them out of the office is like dealing with the Tar Baby. Worse, they return before their next appointment, and telephone for help in between, often interminably. The doctor's responsiveness and patience is met with effusive, flattering gratitude, especially at first. This **exaggerated gratitude is an early clue.** Initially pleasurable, this soon sours. At best, the demands become wearing beyond endurance; and they escalate to insatiability. Unless the pattern is interrupted, rejection is inevitable, to which they respond with deeply hurt feelings. This may manipulate the doctor to reinitiate the cycle out of guilt, making it worse the next go-around.

The problem, of course, is bottomless dependency, unleashed by the illness. It is neither possible nor useful to fulfill this demand. Once the problem is recognized, the doctor must **set clear limits, kindly but absolutely firmly,** reiterated as often as necessary. Specific rules must be set about extracurricular calls and appointments. **Concomitantly the doctor must let the patient know he does care and will provide continuing support** by saying so, and by offering a **specific** appointment at an appropriate interval.

The Malignant "Crock"

Here the problem is that the somatic symptoms themselves arise out of psychopathology, and are vastly out of proportion or unrelated to the somatic pathology. These patients suffer from a *somatization disorder,* a serious, chronic psychiatric condition. (Hence a detailed description is provided elsewhere; see Chapter 14.) To summarize, illness and medical care have become their way of life. They experience multiple, fluctuating, intractable symptoms in multiple systems, some of which arise as somatic or psychological side effects to the treatment they insist upon. They seek out consultations and surgery. Also termed "manipulative help rejectors," in reality they do not reject help, just its effectiveness—as they are eager to report. The doctor's emotional problems are twofold. Such patients remain with him like an albatross, never getting well, and provoking frustration and a sense of failure. They serve also as a source of continuing anxiety, lest another, more treatable medical diagnosis has been missed, originally or intercurrently. But once their psychiatric problem is recognized, they can be managed with reasonable effectiveness and comfort (as outlined also in Chapter 14).

The Intimidating–Demanding Patient

The claims for care by this type of patient are neither stickily clinging nor at all flattering. They are expressed as angry, dissatisfied demands for better treatment; nasty, supercilious complaints; and threats—implied or overt—as to what will befall the doctor should he fail. Paranoid is an apt descriptor, though misplaced if used as a diagnosis, and perilous if overheard. Their sense of need is every bit as intense as the previous groups. They are frightened to death by their illness and by the possibility that the doctor will not take care of them. But rather than wheedle, seduce and cling, they try to extract care via intimidation and domination. These devices are designed not only to satisfy their excessive needs, but to obscure from their own awareness that these needs are present. Rather, they imply that care is their due, that they are "entitled"—more than entitled, for they have been abused. The doctor's usual reaction is one of rage mixed with fear. He would like to tell the patient off, and send him off; but dare not, lest the threats be carried out. In the hospital, the entire staff may be terrorized.

There is no easy answer to dealing with these people. The best approach begins with **acknowledging justified complaints.** As with most "paranoid" accusations, there is always at least a grain of truth to these. Defensiveness merely adds fuel to the fire. Arguments are fruitless. Even the complaint that the doctor has not made him well can be acknowledged; the frustration of being ill is familiar enough. The underlying insecurity is never confronted, however. **While accepting the angry feelings, the doctor indicates that the patient's behavior is interfering with treatment,** while overtly reaffirming his commitment to provide that treatment. Finally, the doctor can **suggest that the patient use his anger in the service of treatment,** by pushing himself to carry out required terrible procedures, working to "lick" the pain or disability, etc.

The Masochistic Borderline Patient

Elsewhere (Chapter 8) the features of the borderline personality disorder are described. These impulsive, inconstant, emotionally volatile people are always difficult to manage. Only so long as the doctor panders to their whims and immediate states of mind do they cooperate. Easily frustrated, they then become depressed or angered. Happily for the nonpsychiatrist, they usually move on to find a "better" doctor.

A particular subgroup of these patients seem **hell-bent on destroying themselves.** As psychiatric patients, they engage in repetitive suicidal acts, preferably in a way that embarrasses their psychiatrist. (One slashed her wrists on the psychiatrist's doorstep, with an appointment card in her purse.) Their behavior, which may include alcohol and drug abuse, often leads to medical problems. However illness develops, they use that condition to pursue their aims to "get even" with a frightening world (including their doctors) by being self-destructive. They are quite willing, indeed eager, to crush themselves as they pull down the walls of the Temple. Temporarily stayed, they raise the ante at the next opportunity. They drink more in the face of varices, overdose with or fail to take their medication, and ignore infections. In the hospital, they pull out IVs and catheters, refuse critical tests, break equipment, and are noisy and demanding. Almost inevitably, their doctors and nurses become furious (which is exactly what they wish). Only by massive self-control, and reaching down to the wellsprings of our compassion, do we avoid simply letting them die, an outcome that is often inevitable despite heroic efforts. When that occurs, we breathe a sigh of secret relief—sometimes not so secret.

Little can be done for these patients, though rarely psychiatric treatment can reverse the process. But recognizing what is happening and coming to terms with the presence of our rage does help. It becomes easier to control; and less likely to make us simultaneously guilty. We can then go about our business of working to prolong their lives as best we can.

Additional Readings

Bibring GL: Psychiatry and medical practice in a general hospital. New Engl J Med 254:366–372, 1956

Groves JE: Taking care of the hateful patient. New Engl J Med 298:883–887, 1978

Kahana RJ, Bibring GL: Personality types in medical management, in Psychiatry and Medical Practice in a General Hospital. Edited by Zinberg NE. New York, International Universities Press, 1964, pp 108–123

Lipsett DR: Medical and psychological characteristics of "crocks." Psychiatr Med 1:15–25, 1970

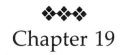

Chapter 19

Compliance

Donald Oken

In recent years it has been "discovered" that few patients accurately pursue all aspects of their prescribed regimens. Why should that surprise us? The most minimal self-examination reveals that we doctors do the same. (Indeed, it is likely that we are among the worst offenders.) At the least, it is hard to remember to do something new and different. When what is required is unpleasant, difficult, or even stressful, there is an even stronger inclination to fail to comply. The wonder is that patients do as well as they do. Yet studies indicate consistently that **doctors seriously underestimate the frequency and magnitude of non-compliance.** At least minor errors or deficiencies in so simple an aspect of treatment as medication taking have been shown to occur about 90% of the time. Once we face squarely that this is commonplace, we can begin to have more tolerance for the patient whom we "catch" in non-compliance, and to develop better techniques for reducing its prevalence. Actually, much is known already about the factors involved and ways to correct these.

Patient and Treatment Factors

Since it is the patient who fails to comply, it is to them the doctor tends to look first as the cause. But it has proved **impossible to establish psychological or social profiles of the poor complier to use as predictors.** A few groups do have demonstrably higher rates of noncompliance: notably the aged, patients with major psychiatric disorders and adolescents. But other patient determinants have been pursued in vain.

At first it was thought that non-middle-class patient groups (and the features which characterize them) could be implicated. It has since become clear that it was the setting which proved to explain class differences, where these initially seemed relevant. "Charity" and clinic settings are conducive to poorer rates of compliance. The same patients who attend these are not poorer compliers when treated in settings which parallel private, middle-class care. The real determinant seems to be the difference in doctors' behaviors and relationships to patients in such settings.

Of course, there are individuals who have a predilection for noncompliance. Evidence of prior irresponsibility, risk taking, denial of illness, self-destructiveness, etc., may give clues. A history of repeated prior noncompliance is a strong predictor. If any of these factors are suspected, the regimen should be kept as simple as possible, with emphasis on treatment that produce evident, observable effects quickly.

Factors in the patient's current life affect compliance. The extent of social supports and the degree to which key others promote the treatment are relevant factors. Compliance decreases in the presence of life stress of any type, especially for treatments altering lifestyle. Clearly, the doctor can serve as an additional source of social support (or stress!).

The **nature of the treatment and the regimen are demonstrably important factors.** Most of these factors, whose validity is obvious, can be simply described.

1. Treatments which involve **changes in lifestyle** (eating, sleeping, working, etc.) have low rates of compliance compared with traditional therapies, such as medications.
2. Among lifestyle changes, those which involve **doing without something** (dieting, smoking, etc.) have lower rates of compliance than those requiring doing something new (e.g., exercise).
3. The **greater the number of different treatments** or medications, the poorer the compliance.
4. The **longer the duration,** the poorer the compliance.
5. The **more frequent or more complex the schedule,** the poorer the compliance. It is best to link schedules to established life routines (bedtimes, mealtimes, etc.) and to schedule different treatments as similarly as possible.
6. The more **complex the method for obtaining the correct dose,** the poorer the compliance. For example, pills requiring halving, or liquids to be measured out are less likely to be taken, or taken accurately. Pills which look alike may be confused.
7. Treatment without immediately **observable effects** are less likely to be continued. Even side effects, if not frightening, promote compliance.

Role of the Doctor in Compliance

The question in compliance is not: "Who is to blame?" but "What can we do to improve it?" To get away from the false lead of blame, "adherence" has been suggested as a substitute term. This also helps avoid the implication that someone is failing to obey "orders." However we name this rose, the point is that the doctor has unique leverage on the situation.

The core of this is the quality of the **doctor–patient relationship.** Within its supportive structure, the patient has infinitely greater faith in the value of the treatment and willingness to pursue it, thereby enhancing its effectiveness also.

Beyond this, the physician's approach to the instructions makes a demonstrable difference. This is not to say that there is one right way. **The approach must be flexibly adapted to the patient.** This includes the flexibility to be rigid for those patients to whom only hard-and-fast, detailed instructions convey that a treatment is valuable (e.g., "Take 2 pills 35 minutes before each meal, with a half-glass of milk."). It is always possible to give a patient some degree of choice, if participation in decision making is crucial to that type of person. ("Would you prefer the injection in your arm or buttock?"; "Would you prefer a larger pill to swallow only once daily or smaller ones several times a day?") With long-standing patients, the doctor usually knows what approach works best. But even with these, **it is essential to take time to find out what the patient wishes (needs) to know.**

Initial instructions should be simple, concrete, and direct, and given without request. This should include information about probable side effects. Foreknowledge of these reduces fearful, angry noncompliance; and when they occur, the doctor's credibility is reinforced and the notion that a powerful therapy is at work is confirmed, enhancing compliance.

This is always followed by giving the patient explicit opportunity to request more information. Some patients do not want to know any more; but they are rare. If no questions are forthcoming, it is best to ask something general like: "Is that entirely clear?"; and then to wait for a response. The patient must have a genuine opportunity to voice requests for information and reassurance. The latter are interdependent. While patients often do wish to know more, the doctor's demonstrated willingness to respond to this may be as important as the information itself.

Explanations are tailored to the style and the content of the questions ("the music along with the words"). The fearfulness of a question may be more relevant than the query itself. Questions cannot be taken at face value and merely answered concretely. One must elicit **the meaning of the inquiry:** the question behind the question. Not only overt feelings, but wording, repetitions, etc., give clues that something else is involved.

involved. A patient expressing concern about side effects may really be anxious as to whether the treatment will work, itself linked to yet more important fears about the illness, or other issues. (One patient expected that his pneumonia was imminently fatal because the rusty sputum it caused recalled the fatal hemoptasis of a tubercular family member. Only after substantial effort to pursue his otherwise unexplained anxious questioning did this real concern emerge.)

Nevertheless, it is also common that a patient simply fails to understand instructions. Anxiety about health promotes poor concentration and confusion, even among intelligent patients. Eager not to "bother" or antagonize the busy doctor, the patient may not request crucial clarifications until given abundant encouragement by the doctor's unhurried interest. Clearly worded written instructions provide a valuable adjunct for later reference. But these never replace the doctor's person, merely supplement it.

When noncompliance is revealed, the reflex reaction is to scold the patient, or paint a picture of dire consequences. These commonsense responses only reflect the doctor's frustration, and undermine the relationship. Neither reaction is effective. If compliance does improve, which is rare, it does so only transiently. (Seeming improvement most likely only reflects the patient's fear now to tell the truth.) Of course, noncompliance should not be ignored. **The doctor indicates his positive concern, and inquires about the reasons in a noncritical way.** Simple explanation, reassurance, or minor changes in the regimen may meet the objections, if the patient is given the comfort to reveal them. Real reasons behind given reasons must have the opportunity for expression. If necessary, compromises are made. The doctor must accept the fact that entrenched behaviors, such as smoking, cannot be given up without great effort or discomfort. If carried out despite this, because of absolute necessity, the doctor must be prepared to treat overt anxiety or depression.

The doctor's person—his relationship to the patient—is the most potent force in the medical armamentarium. It is directly therapeutic; it augments the effects of all other treatments; and it is the most effective device for enhancing that aspect of cooperation we term compliance.

Additional Readings

Blackwell B: The drug defaulter. Clin Pharm Ther 13:841–848, 1972

Christenson DB: Drug-taking compliance: A review and synthesis. Health Serv Res 13(2):171–187, 1978

Davis MS: Variations in patients' compliance with doctors' orders: Analyses of congruence between survey responses and results of empirical investigations. J Med Educ 41:1037–1048, 1966

Kasl S: Socio-psychological characteristics associated with behaviors which reduce cardiovascular risk, in Applying Behavioral Science to Cardiovascular Risk, Proceedings of a Conference. Edited by Enelow A, Henderson JB. New York, American Heart Association, 1975, pp 173–190

Marston MV: Compliance with medical regimens: A review of the literature. Nurs Res 19:312–323, 1970

Patient Compliance. Edited by Lasagna L. Mt. Kisco, N.Y., Futura, 1976

PART VI

TREATMENT

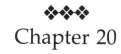

Chapter 20

Practical Psychotherapy

Magnus Lakovics

A primary distinction must be made between general psychotherapeutic management and formal psychotherapy as treatment. Psychotherapeutic management entails establishment of a good doctor–patient relationship and an approach which capitalizes upon several potent nonspecific factors inherent in the "healing" influence. Psychotherapy entails specialized techniques which are designed to deal with specific problems. These are complex and require substantial training to master and utilize.

A good doctor embodies such qualities as empathy, acceptance, kindness, compassion, integrity, willingness to listen, and maturity. The ability to manifest these qualities with an emotionally disturbed, critically ill, difficult or dying patient in stressful environments such as the emergency room, ICU, or ward is central to establishing and maintaining a good doctor–patient relationship. This relationship alone has powerful positive effects on the patient's attitudes toward his illness and treatment. A closer look at the psychological features of this relationship reveals that the healing influence is determined by several factors. Utilization of these as principles guiding treatment characterizes the effective therapist, regardless of his particular "orientation" or the type of treatment being used. These include: a confiding relationship, a rationale to explain the cause of the patient's problem, new information, and alternative solutions; arousal of hope and facilitating success experiences, which enhance the patient's self-esteem; and facilitating emotional arousal. Many physicians intuitively utilize these principles in daily practice. Nevertheless, the ability to focus and actively utilize them can result in substantially more productive psychotherapeutic management (without four years of specialty training in psychiatry).

General Principles of Psychotherapeutic Management
A Confiding Relationship

To confide in a person requires **trust**. Trust in varying degrees is accorded to all doctors as a function of their professional role in our culture. However, many psychiatric patients and others have often had traumatic and conflicted experiences in early childhood with their first major relationships (parents). As a consequence, their level of general trust often is diminished. Even where this is not the case, discussion of intimate relationships, fears, hopes, painful feelings and sexual life, etc. is often embarrassing and difficult. To maximize the patient's ability to confide, the physician needs to provide time and privacy, to have a nonjudgmental, noncritical attitude, and to be willing to listen to anything without excessive anxiety or embarrassment himself. The confiding relationship also has a responsibility attached to it: to have what is said remain confidential. At times, this may mean assuring the patient of this directly by indicating that records are kept locked or that very personal details (as distinguished from clinical details) are not recorded. Confidentiality is also transmitted nonverbally as well. Closing the door (or lowering one's voice, when the setting is public) conveys much. In contrast, a physician overheard talking in the hallway about another patient undermines himself.

An Etiological Rationale

It is the nature of being human to want some rational explanation for an event, especially one which is troubling. Illness is certainly no exception. One important aspect of this, particularly with psychiatric patients, is that mastery of problems ("cure") often depends on knowing their causes or origins for resolution. The patient needs a basis for understanding **why they have occurred.** Thus, a mutual discussion of reasons underlying development of a problem can substantially contribute to achieving relief. For example, if the object of fear can be identified with a panicky patient, this may be all that is necessary. For someone who seeks attention for back pain, sensitively discussing the tensions of his current life may preclude the need to prescribe medication.

Such a discussion with the physician emphasizes the patient's active participation in the treatment process rather than promoting passivity. It also encourages respect for the physician by giving an indication of his competence (which presumably rests on having a rationale for treatment), thus enhancing the relationship.

Having Alternatives

Illness (unless minor and common such as a cold) is a signal to see the doctor. When a patient does, he has chosen one alternative which he feels will provide a solution to the problem presented. He expects the physician to help. With straightforward, simple problems, the physician can provide a ready solution (e.g., sewing up a laceration). Similarly, even with more complex problems, patients expect the same. Many times they have tried other alternatives but have met with failure (e.g., dietary changes for chronic fatigue). When these alternatives have not worked, their last resort may be their physician.

This is common with many psychiatric problems. Patients attempt changes in lifestyle, relationships, employment, etc. before seeking professional help. They may even attempt self-injury as a solution or a means to one. This demonstrates how fully they have exhausted their resources and now must rely on someone else with more knowledge. Expectations can be quite high.

With psychiatric patients, the physician can supply many alternatives such as medication, referral, and hospitalization. However, one very important option sometimes ignored is the **mutual exploration of the problems without having an answer.** The exploration may reveal some sources of the problem, provide emotional support, stimulate further exploration, and raise hopes. Because of high expectations about his own performance, the physician often feels pressured to provide specific solutions, and if he cannot he may mistakenly dismiss the patient out of frustration. With many psychiatric problems, there may be no specific answer or solution. In fact, the process of exploration may be one of the first alternatives which directly and indirectly demonstrates that others may be possible.

Arousal of Hope

With all illness, hope is essential for seeking out and continuing with treatment, and in itself, provides relief. A time-tested way of instilling hope is through **reassurance.** Reassurance can be nonverbal and verbal. Nonverbal reassurance occurs through the attitude and manner conveyed by the doctor. A realistic, optimistic attitude coupled with an empathic, knowledgeable, and sensitive manner raise expectations and hopes. Many times with psychiatric patients reassurance is complex and not easy to do. Although attitude and manner remain the same, verbal reassurance can be tricky. This problem arises because their overt complaints sometimes do not reflect their underlying concerns, fears and conflicts. For example, a patient with a major depression may feel he is going to die and may react with more depression when reassured he is healthy. The response is understandable considering his condition and the underlying feelings. Depression often results from poor self-esteem, guilt, or anger turned at the self. He may actually have an unconscious wish to die. Good health may only prolong his misery. Reassuring this patient that he's not going to die may have the opposite effect than that intended. On the other hand, delving into some negative feelings he has about himself, recommending referral, and being cautiously optimistic may provide the reassurance which allows him to have some hope and to comply with the referral.

Facilitating Success Experiences

Psychiatric disorders vary in the degree of functional incapacity. Some patients are totally disabled (e.g., severe degenerative dementia); others can maintain a high level of function in some areas but show deficiency in others (e.g., phobic neurosis). Regardless of the degree of functional incapacity, it is distressing, and, if allowed to continue, can further lower morale. Facilitating success experiences even to a minor degree is necessary to improve and maintain functioning as well as encouraging continued involvement in treatment. An essential ingredient of this is a **realistic evaluation of the patient's areas of functional incapacity.** If the evaluation is unrealistic and expectations are too great, this leads to failure experiences. The failure experience in turn can lead to noncompliance, frustration, deterioration, and loss of faith and trust in the physician. On the other hand, if the condition is appraised realistically and recommendations take into account strengths and weaknesses, the likelihood of being successful in reaching expected goals is greater. This further enhances self-esteem which leads to further gain.

A key in all of this is discussing the felt incapacities and proposed treatment plan in an open and frank manner with the patient. This also results in gaining more information, since it may be the only way to tell if the patient is using defenses (e.g., denial) that preclude a successful appraisal of difficulties, compliance with treatment recommendations, and referral. For example, a mistakenly held belief about some psychiatric problems is that they can simply be reversed by strength of will. Statements like: "Don't fight with your husband. You can stop it if you try. Don't think about it. You have so many things going for you. Don't be depressed, it's normal. Don't worry about it, etc." highlight this approach. Because the source of difficulty is often unconscious, this misleading approach results in making the patient feel guilty and worse.

On the other hand, realistic recognition of the dilemma can lead to progress. Thus, statements like: "You feel as if it is out of your control. What are you prevented from doing because you feel this way? Tell me what you feel you can do, etc." can be helpful in expanding the discussion, appraising the felt incapacity and developing a plan which is consistent with the patient's abilities and wishes. Another common error is responding to manipulation when a patient should be able to function in a particular area but is seen as being weaker than he actually is. This occurs through gaining the overwhelming sympathy of the doctor. A group particularly prone to this are those who have had a serious illness and never seem to recover (e.g., cardiac neurosis). In this case, realistic evaluation of capacities again is helpful. Rather than providing sympathy, the doctor can firmly and sensitively develop a plan which emphasizes strengths not just weaknesses.

Facilitating Emotional Arousal

Human beings often tend not to be actively conscious of many feeling states. Psychiatric patients in particular share this, but also suffer from repressed feelings, inability to control feeling states (affective disorders), having mixed-up thoughts and feelings (schizophrenic disorders), and being unable to come to terms with feelings about stressful life events (adjustment disorders). In each of these situations, facilitating emotional arousal is beneficial and necessary to obtain history, establish rapport, and provide support and relief. However, as with all techniques, it can also increase anxiety by setting aside defenses which have kept a precarious balance within mental functioning (e.g., delving too much into the feeling states of psychotic patients).

Facilitating emotional arousal requires that a confiding relationship be established (as previously discussed). Once this is done, **ventilation of feelings** *(catharsis)* is possible. This may sound easy, but many patients may not be able to ventilate because of embarrassment, shame, and fear. Defenses such as repression, denial, displacement, etc. may also prevent them from talking about conflicted feelings. This requires an open-ended approach (see Chapter 1) with fewer "checklist" questions. It is also important to be accepting rather than confronting or challenging. One precaution is that too much ventilation can also be harmful. The best way to avoid this is to gently guide the conversation, following cues from the patient. If he is very unwilling to discuss something, it may be best to leave it alone for the time being. Later, the reluctance may diminish. An additional possibility is to ask about the reluctance itself.

Another important principle is to **comment on feelings rather than content.** For example, a patient may talk about the death of a loved one in discussing past history. A comment such as "it must have made you feel pretty bad" will elicit more information but also can be supportive.

Once confidence is established, ventilation occurs and feelings are elaborated, and a more intense relationship develops. The involvement may give rise to problems as well as benefits. Because of this intensity, positive or negative feelings out of proportion to the circumstances can result in the doctor or the patient. Anticipation and awareness of the indicators of this occurrence is necessary. These indicators are things like unexplained, irrational anger, excessive dependency, or erotic fantasies. If they have developed and become unmanageable, an informal consultation with a psychiatrist colleague may be useful or referral may become necessary.

Formal Psychotherapeutic Treatment

Although psychotherapeutic treatment is based on verbal and nonverbal communication, there are a vast array of techniques from hypnosis, behavior therapy, family therapy, group therapy, and classical psychoanalysis. Many of these techniques are very specific and specialized. For example, systematic desensitization, a type of behavior therapy, is useful in the treatment of phobias. Hypnosis can be very useful in pain management. Family therapy may be essential in management and treatment of the schizophrenic. Classical psychoanalysis is effective for symptomatic neuroses. A psychotherapeutic approach which is commonly applied to a broad spectrum of psychiatric problems (from adjustment reactions to schizophrenia) is psychodynamically based individual psychotherapy. A fair generalization can be made that patients referred to a general psychiatrist, if treated with psychotherapy, will be treated this way with the addition of other therapies (e.g., psychotropics, ECT, group, and family therapy) as indicated.

In dynamically based individual psychotherapy, the therapist usually meets for 45 minutes to an hour once or twice weekly for several months or in many cases several years. The therapist and patient agree to basic ground rules in the first few sessions. The patient is asked to say whatever comes to mind. The therapist assures complete confidentiality. Sessions are scheduled on a regular basis. The ground rules are designed to create an atmosphere in which the patient will feel free to discuss intimate problems, to allow affective expression, and also to more or less (depending on the degree of psychopathology) develop a relationship with the therapist which may have characteristics similar to other important relationships in the patient's life (transference). This usually involves significant others such as mother, father, siblings, spouse, etc. The therapist must also be alert to development of emotional responses in himself which may be reactions to the patient's conflict or may originate from the therapist's own past and emotional conflicts *(countertransferences)*. The aim is to uncover unconscious conflicts operative in life resulting in symptoms, unpleasant feelings, and interpersonal difficulties. At times the therapist may be judiciously supportive and not necessarily delve deep, particularly in psychotic patients. Other aims of therapy may be to alleviate and eliminate symptoms, change unwanted personality characteristics, and assist in interpersonal functioning.

Awareness by the physician that psychotherapy is a slow, involved, and intensive process is necessary so that misunderstanding does not occur when referral is made and progress is not quickly seen. In addition, the need for confidentiality sometimes is also misunderstood by family members and the referring physician as indifference, secretiveness, and lack of consideration. It is helpful for the referring physician to inform and educate family members about the nature of psychotherapeutic treatment when they look to their trusted doctor to explain why progress is not occurring after several sessions and wonder why no contact and information is provided by the psychiatrist.

Conclusion

Principles of psychotherapeutic management and treatment within the sphere of medical practice have many applications. Some key concepts and their usefulness in practice have been discussed. Utilization of psychotherapeutic management principles is essential in the formation of a working doctor–patient relationship, eliciting history of less obvious or underlying problems, and understanding and/or dealing with untoward or unusual reactions, adaptations, to psychiatric or other medical illness. Finally, it is important for the physician to have a general understanding of what formal psychotherapy entails and to inform patients and family members about what can be expected from it.

Additional Readings

An Introduction to the Psychotherapies. Edited by Bloch S. Oxford, Oxford University Press, 1979 (This is a good introductory text for the nonpsychiatrist discussing different specific therapies as well as the general approach.)

Frank J: Therapeutic factors in psychotherapy. Am J Psychotherapy 25:350–361, 1971

Karasu TB: Psychotherapies: An overview. Am J Psychiatry 134:851–863, 1977

Strupp HH: On the technology of psychotherapy. Arch Gen Psychiatry 26:270–278, 1972

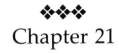

Chapter 21

Psychopharmacology

Donald M. Pirodsky

In a little over a quarter of a century, psychopharmacological agents have become the most frequently prescribed group of drugs in the world. Paralleling the rapid advances in psychopharmacology has been an ever-increasing body of knowledge in biological psychiatry.

Antipsychotic (Neuroleptic) Agents

Also called *major tranquilizers,* that term leads to confusion in thinking of these drugs as being similar in action to sedatives or "minor tranquilizers," which are qualitatively entirely different. Table 1 lists all of the significant agents, providing both generic and trade names together with their ususal oral dosage ranges and relative potency on a weight basis.

Indications for Use

The antipsychotics are powerful drugs. Their use should be reserved for **major** psychiatric disorders. They are useful also for certain serious medical and neurological problems. Their main indications are:

Schizophrenia. **This is their primary indication;** and includes both acute and chronic schizophrenia. Improvement in both the thought disorder and degree of agitation or withdrawal is usually noted; they calm agitated schizophrenics and activate those who are withdrawn.

Table 1. Equivalent Doses and Usual Daily Dose Ranges of Oral Forms of
Antipsychotic Agents

Generic Name	Trade Name	Approximate Equivalent Dose (mg)	Usual Daily Dose Range (mg/day)	
			Acute	Maintenance
Phenothiazines				
Aliphatic				
Chlorpromazine	Thorazine[a]	100[b]	300–1600	100–400
Triflupromazine	Vesprin	25	75–150	25–100
Piperidine				
Mesoridazine	Serentil	50	150–400	50–200
Piperacetazine	Quide	10	40–160	20–50
Thioridazine	Mellaril[a]	100	300–800	100–400
Piperazine				
Acetophenazine	Tindal	20	60–120	40–80
Butaperazine	Repoise	10	30–100	10–40
Carphenazine	Proketazine	25	75–400	25–150
Fluphenazine	{ Prolixin / Permitil	2	6–60	2–8
Perphenazine	Trilafon	8	16–64	8–24
Prochlorperazine	Compazine	15	50–150	20–60
Trifluoperazine	Stelazine	5	15–60	5–15
Thioxanthenes				
Chlorprothixene	Taractan	100	300–600	75–400
Thiothixene	Navane	5	15–60	6–30
Butyrophenones				
Haloperidol	Haldol	2	6–100	2–8
Dihydroindolones				
Molindone	Moban Lidone	10	40–225	15–60
Dibenzoxazepines				
Loxapine	Loxitane Daxolin	15	50–250	20–75

[a]Chlorpromazine and Thioridazine are also available generically.
[b]100 mg of chlorpromazine is set as the base for comparison.

Schizophreniform disorder is the name now applied in the third edition
of the *Diagnostic and Statistical manual* (DSM III) of the American
Psychiatric Association to illnesses indistinguishable from schizophrenia but of less than 6 months' duration. *Brief reactive psychosis*
(another new term) is similar, but even briefer and clearly stress
related. What is said here about the treatment of acute schizophrenia
applies to both.

Mania. Antipsychotics often are needed to control acute manic states
in manic–depressive disorders. Although lithium is the primary

treatment for mania, it has a slow onset of action; and a neuroleptic may need to be given concurrently until the acute episode is under control.

Organic mental disorders. Although not the primary treatment of these disorders (see Chapter 4), antipsychotics are useful to control agitation, excitement, or belligerent behavior associated with confusion and thought disorganization.

Depression. Antipsychotics are not the drugs of choice in treating depression (tricyclic antidepressants are), and **can make some depressions worse.** But at times a combination of a tricyclic and a neuroleptic is indicated for psychotic and severely agitated depressions, and is more effective than the tricyclic alone.

Psychoses and behavioral problems associated with mental retardation. Antipsychotics often are a useful adjunct in the treatment of those retarded patients who manifest severe self-abusive behavior, unprovoked aggressive behavior, autistic-like behaviors (repetitive, stereotyped, self-stimulatory behaviors), or uncontrollable hyperactivity.

Gilles de la Tourette's syndrome. This rare disorder is responsive to haloperidol.

Chemical and Pharmacologic Properties

All known antipsychotic drugs block CNS postsynaptic dopamine receptors. This is their presumed mechanism of action. The receptor blockade in the basal ganglia produces extrapyramidal side effects.

In general, the antipsychotics are well absorbed orally (especially in liquid form), reaching peak plasma levels in 2 to 4 hours. IM injection results in complete absorption, producing plasma levels approximately four times that of equivalent oral doses (e.g., 50 mg IM of chlorpromazine = 200 mg orally). Their plasma half-life is long, roughly 12 to 24 hours; hence they need be given only once or twice a day.

Phenothiazines

There are three subgroups based on differences in the side chain of the phenothiazine nucleus.

ALIPHATIC PHENOTHIAZINES

These are strongly sedating and anticholinergic and have significant antiemetic effects. They are also potent alpha-adrenergic blockers; and therefore can produce profound postural hypotension. They produce extrapyramidal syndromes less frequently than the piperazine pheno-thiazines.

Chlorpromazine frequently causes postural hypotension, especially when given IM. No more than 100 mg IM should be given at one time. IM chlorpromazine is also very irritating.

Triflupromazine is about four times as potent by weight as chlorprom-azine.

PIPERIDINE PHENOTHIAZINES

Thioridazine is the **most anticholinergic** of all antipsychotics, hence least likely to produce extrapyramidal side effects. It is about as sedating as chlorpromazine, and also produces postural hypotension secondary to peripheral adrenergic blockade. That effect also can inhibit or produce retrograde ejaculation. It is the only phenothiazine without an antiemetic effect. Because of the risk of developing pigmentary retinopathy at doses over 800 mg/day, this **dose ceiling** has been established (the only antip-sychotic with an absolute dose limit). Thioridazine is the antipsychotic most often associated with EKG abnormalities. It is not available in a parenteral form.

Mesoridazine, which comes in an injectable form, is about twice as potent as thioridazine (of which it is a metabolite). But pigmentary ret-inopathy has **not** been associated with its use; and EKG changes are less common. It is strongly sedative.

Piperacetazine resembles the piperazines in structure. Thus, its actions are similar to that group.

PIPERAZINE PHENOTHIAZINES

These have the strongest antiemetic effects and are the most potent group on a mg per mg basis. Sedation, postural hypotension, and an-ticholinergic effects are less prominent. They are the worst offenders in terms of **extrapyramidal side effects.**

Acetophenazine produces the fewest extrapyramidal side effects of this subgroup. It may be useful in patients who tolerate such symptoms poorly.

Perphenazine also produces fewer extrapyramidal symptoms than other piperazines. It is the only antipsychotic marketed in combination with a tricyclic antidepressant (amitriptyline). When used clinically, the two drugs are generally prescribed separately to give more flexibility in ar-riving at the best dosage of each. Fixed combination preparations may be suitable for maintenance treatment, once the dosage has been estab-lished. Because of the strong anticholinergic properties of tricyclics, ex-trapyramidal side effects are infrequent with this combination.

Fluphenazine is **the only antipsychotic in a long-acting injectable form.** There are two such preparations available: the enanthate (effective for 1 to 3 weeks), and the decanoate (effective for 2 to 4 weeks). Both contain 25 mg/cc of fluphenazine. These are useful for maintenance therapy but not recommended for initial treatment. They are invaluable for patients who are unreliable about taking medication, or who absorb oral agents poorly. The main side effects with these depot preparations are extrapyramidal symptoms, especially acute dystonic reactions. These generally occur 1 to 5 days after injection, and are more common with the enanthate.

Prochlorperazine is used primarily for its strong antiemetic effect.

Other Neuroleptics

BUTRYOPHENONES

This class of neuroleptics is unrelated chemically to the phenothiazines. However, their pharmacologic properties closely resemble the piperazine phenothiazines. They are strong antiemetics, have a high relative potency, and cause minimal sedation. Their anticholinergic and alpha-adrenergic blocking effects are also minimal. They have a strong tendency to evoke **extrapyramidal reactions.**

Haloperidol is the only butryophenone approved for use as an antipsychotic in this country. It is an excellent drug for treatment of acute psychoses. Some authors recommend its use for rapid tranquilization of acute schizophrenic patients, a procedure where it is given IM every 30 to 60 minutes until improvement occurs. It is less irritating IM than chlorpromazine, and also much less likely to produce a serious hypotensive reaction.

Droperidol is used primarily as an anesthetic premedication and induction agent in this country. It has been reported to be effective in managing excited states from a variety of causes; and in Europe is used for its antipsychotic properties.

THIOXANTHENES

These closely resemble the phenothiazines structurally and pharmacologically.

Chlorprothixene is the thioxanthene analog of chlorpromazine, and has similar properties.

Thiothixene is one of the least sedating agents. Its chemical structure and pharmacologic actions are similar to those of the piperazine phenothiazines. Akathisia is its main side effect.

DIBENZOXAZEPINES

Loxapine is the representative of this new class of neuroleptics. It is sedating, and frequently produces extrapyramidal reactions. Alpha-adrenergic blockade is reported to be low to moderate, as are anticholinergic effects. In general, clinicians reserve the use of the newer anti-psychotic agents (molindone and loxapine) for patients who are refractory to, or who cannot tolerate the more established drugs.

DIHYDROINDOLONES

Molindone is the only drug of this class presently in use. Although its structure is unrelated to the other classes of antipsychotic agents, its clinical effects are similar to those of the piperazine phenothiazines, haloperidol and thiothixene. It produces a moderate degree of sedation and alpha-adrenergic blocking. However, its most frequent side effect is some type of extrapyramidal reaction, most often akathisia.

Guidelines for Clinical Use

TREATMENT OF SCHIZOPHRENIA

Hospital treatment by a psychiatrist is required for acute psychoses, except in extraordinary circumstances.

Make an **accurate diagnosis** before initiating treatment. Be sure that the symptoms are known to be relieved by the medication.

The choice of a specific agent should, when possible, be based on the patient's prior drug response history: one effective for a prior episode should be tried first. If this is the first use, the choice should be based on the family drug response history. If neither guideline is available, the choice is often based on the side effects produced. For example, sedation may be desirable in an agitated schizophrenic but unwanted in one who is withdrawn. Hypotensive side effects would be undesirable in a patient on antihypertensive medication or in the elderly.

Potency is not to be confused with efficacy. Although the drugs vary in potency on a weight basis, all are effective when given in **equivalent doses.** The physician should pick one or two drugs from each of the subgroups of phenothiazines, and one from the other chemical classes, and become fully familiar with their effects.

Treatment of a newly diagnosed schizophrenic should be initiated with a small test dose to check for any adverse effect. After 2 hours, one begins increasing the dose into the effective antipsychotic range (see Table 1). The rate of increase depends on the clinical condition of the patient. The dose then is increased gradually every 2 to 3 days until an adequate therapeutic response is achieved, or troublesome side effects intervene. This is generally done within a 6-week period; but patients with exacerbations of chronic schizophrenia may need a 3-month period before response should be judged. The dose ranges given in Table 1 are usual ranges; but the individual needs of each patient must be taken into account. For young, acutely agitated schizophrenics, the starting dose could be higher and the dosage increased more rapidly. For older patients or those less agitated, the reverse is true. However, insufficient dosage may be one reason for failure to respond.

Divided doses usually are best initially. This minimizes the impact of side effects and allows better titration of dose. Once a therapeutic dose is established, the frequency can be reduced. All antipsychotics are long-acting and need be given no more than one to two times per day. A single bedtime dose often is feasible. This increases compliance and reduces side effects. If a divided dose schedule is appropriate, the majority of the dose (e.g., two-thirds) can be given at bedtime. But elderly patients may not be able to tolerate a single large dose, and require a t.i.d. or q.i.d. schedule. Satisfactory improvement can be expected in 75% or more of newly admitted patients. The first signs of response generally are in the behavior and sleep pattern. Later, improvement in the thought disorder is noted. Although specific antipsychotic effects may be seen in as little as 2 days, optimal benefit may take 6 weeks or longer.

Once improvement has occurred and stabilized (generally 4 to 12 weeks) one should consider decreasing the dose. (For schizophreniform disorders and acute reactive psychoses, this period may be much shorter.) This should be tapered gradually over a period of weeks, as too rapid a reduction may cause relapse. The eventual maintenance dose should be the minimum amount that retains therapeutic gains and allows the patient to function best. This may be roughly one-third to one-fifth the peak dose, but patients vary greatly.

Maintenance medication for an initial schizophrenic episode may be discontinued after 6 to 8 months, assuming the remission is stable. (Again, shorter for schizophreniform and acute reactive psychoses.) For a second schizophrenic episode, maintenance may be required for 2 years. With more episodes, it may be needed indefinitely. Chronic schizophrenics should be maintained on the **lowest possible dose** that will keep their symptoms in remission; and **periodic attempts should be made to discontinue the drugs** altogether. Many chronic schizophrenics maintained on low doses may be getting little benefit from the drugs, and may be discontinued safely.

Inadequate response suggests the need for switching to another antipsychotic. If a newly diagnosed schizophrenic does not respond well to maximally tolerated doses within 6 weeks (3 months for a chronic schizophrenic), he should be considered refractory. If so, he should be switched to a more potent drug of the same class, or to a drug in another class. For example, a patient refractory to chlorpromazine could be tried on fluphenazine, haloperidol, or thiothixene, but not thioridazine. Before deciding that a patient is refractory, be sure that the lack of response is not due to a failure to ingest or absorb the medication. This may be checked by giving a short course of IM administration.

Polypharmacy should be avoided. The use of two or more antipsychotic agents concurrently has **not** been shown to be effective, and increases the risk of drug interactions and side effects.

Antiparkinsonian agents should not be prescribed routinely, but only to treat extrapyramidal symptoms, should they occur. They should be used as little and for as short a period of time as possible; and discontinued within 3 to 4 months. Less than 10% of patients will require these drugs thereafter.

Guidelines for Use in Other Disorders

Antipsychotic drugs need be used only briefly in delirium, due to its reversible nature. In mania, their use may be discontinued when the patient becomes stabilized on lithium. In the treatment of agitation associated with dementia in the elderly, they are used in lower doses; and those with fewer cardiovascular side effects are better tolerated. (Haloperidol 1 to 9 mg/day is often effective.) Psychoses and behavioral problems associated with mental retardation may require doses of antipsychotics similar to those used to treat schizophrenia. The minimal effective dose should be used; and the drug should be tapered and discontinued periodically to determine if it is still required. In the treatment of Gilles de la Tourette's syndrome with haloperidol, dosage is increased until the symptoms are controlled, and then gradually reduced to a maintenance level.

Side Effects

As previously noted, the choice of neuroleptic often is based on the side effects it produces. In general, the low dose (high potency by weight) agents have more extrapyramidal side effects, but are less prone to cause hypotension or sedation; whereas the reverse is true for the higher dose drugs.

OVERSEDATION

This is common with the aliphatic and piperidine phenothiazines, chlorprothixene, and loxapine. It does diminish over time without reduction in dose, and its impact can be minimized by use of a single bedtime dose.

EXTRAPYRAMIDAL REACTIONS

These are of three different types; and are produced more commonly by the piperazine phenothiazines, haloperidol, thiothixene, molindone, and loxapine.

Acute dystonic reactions are muscle spasms, most commonly involving the neck, trunk, face, and eyes. Clinically, they may present as a torticollis (neck muscles), hyperextension of the trunk, facial grimacing or tics, dysphagia, or an oculogyric crisis. These appear suddenly, generally within the first 7 to 10 days of treatment. They are more common in young males. They can be very frightening; but can be rapidly reversed by an IM or IV injection of one of the **antiparkinsonian agents** listed in Table 2. An oral antiparkinsonian agent then can be given for several days until the risk of developing another reaction diminishes. Treatment with antipsychotics need not be interrupted.

Parkinsonism presents much like the idiopathic form. It generally occurs between the first and fourth weeks of treatment, and is more common in older patients. It responds well to oral antiparkinsonian agents. A temporary lowering of the dose of the neuroleptic may help alleviate symptoms. At times *akinesia* may be the predominant feature of parkinsonism, and can be confused with psychotic withdrawal or depression.

Akathisia is a motor restlessness, often observed as pacing or fidgeting. It generally occurs 2 to 6 weeks after treatment. The danger is that it **may be misdiagnosed as psychotic agitation.** It is the most difficult extrapyramidal reaction to treat, but may respond to a reduction in dose. Antiparkinsonian agents may be helpful; but at times a switch of antipsychotic drug is necessary.

All of the antiparkinsonian agents listed in Table 2, except amantadine, have potent anticholinergic effects. Amantadine, a dopamine agonist, is, therefore, the drug of choice when one wishes to avoid anticholinergic side effects. These agents are long-acting and can be given once or twice daily. Several are available in parenteral form.

TARDIVE DYSKINESIA (TD)

TD is a late-appearing extrapyramidal syndrome manifested by rhythmical, involuntary, persistent movements of the tongue, lips, and facial

TABLE 2. Commonly Used Antiparkinsonian Drugs[a]

Generic Name	Trade Name	Usual Daily Dose Range (mg/day)
Anticholinergic agents		
Benztropine[b]	Cogentin	1–6
Biperiden[b]	Akineton	2–6
Diphenhydramine[b]	Benadryl	25–100
Procyclidine	Kemadrin	6–20
Trihexyphenidyl	Artane, Tremin	2–15
Dopamine agonist		
Amantadine	Symmetrel	100–300

[a]Note: Diphenhydramine is also available generically.
[b]Available in IM and IV preparations for acute dystonic reactions.

muscles. Choreoathetoid movements of the limbs (particularly the fingers and toes) and trunk also occur. In general, TD occurs in patients who have been on high doses of antipsychotics for long periods of time; however, it can occur within a few months. Paradoxically, it often first appears after the medication has been reduced or stopped. Antiparkinsonian drugs are of no benefit and often exacerbate the symptoms. If it is recognized early enough and the antipsychotic medication is slowly reduced and discontinued, it will often remit. However, it can be permanent. **Because there is no effective treatment currently, the key to decreasing the incidence of this serious syndrome is prevention and early detection.** Older patients, particularly women, appear to be at greater risk, although it can occur at any age. All of the antipsychotic agents can produce this disorder. None appears to be safer than the others.

ANTICHOLINERGIC SIDE EFFECTS

These include dry mouth, constipation, urinary hesitancy, blurred near vision, and tachycardia. These are often not serious, and tend to decrease over time. In rare instances, paralytic ileus, infection of a paralyzed bladder, or exacerbation of untreated glaucoma can occur.

ORTHOSTATIC (POSTURAL) HYPOTENSION

This results from alpha-adrenergic blockade. Usually simple postural management techniques suffice. In very severe cases, a pure alpha-stimulator, such as norepinephrine, can be used—not epinephrine, which is also a beta-adrenergic stimulator, and may worsen the problem.

MISCELLANEOUS SIDE EFFECTS

Cardiac toxicity and sudden death have been reported rarely with the phenothiazines. These drugs prolong ventricular repolarization and thus enhance the likelihood of developing a reentry arrhythmia, the probable mechanism in sudden death. Patients with preexisting cardiac problems are at greater risk. The most common EKG changes are prolongation of the Q-T interval, lowering of the S-T segment, and flattening and inversion of the T-wave.

Agranulocytosis and leukopenia occur with the phenothiazines, particularly the aliphatics and piperidines. Agranulocytosis is serious but very rare. It is an idiosyncratic reaction, not related to dosage; and is usually seen in the early weeks of treatment. Elderly women appear most susceptible. Since it occurs abruptly, routine monitoring of the blood count is of no aid. If a patient develops a sore throat, fever, or infection, the drug should be discontinued and a white count obtained immediately. Leukopenia is more common, often transient, and usually of no clinical significance.

Cholestatic jaundice has become an increasingly rare side effect of phenothiazines, with chlorpromazine most frequently implicated. It is a sensitivity reaction, with most cases occurring during the early weeks of treatment. Though generally mild and self-limited, it warrants switching to another class of drugs.

Metabolic and endocrine effects are most often associated with the low-potency phenothiazines. Weight gain can be pronounced. Delayed ovulation and menstruation, amenorrhea, and galactorrhea have been reported, most often with chronic treatment. Gynecomastia, impotence, and decreased libido may be seen in men.

Skin and eye effects have been associated primarily with chlorpromazine and thioridazine. Most serious is the *retinitis pigmentosa* associated with thioridazine, which can produce an **irreversible** loss of vision. Corneal and lens opacities have been reported with prolonged high doses of chlorpromazine. These rarely impair vision and gradually disappear after the drug is stopped. Pigment deposition in the skin following prolonged, high doses of chlorpromazine result in a bluish-gray discoloration over exposed areas. Photosensitivity is also most often associated with chlorpromazine; severe sunburn can result from minimal exposure to sunlight. This can be prevented by avoiding exposure and using protective sunscreen preparations. Maculopapular rashes may occur, but are usually transient; because cross-sensitivity is rare, another drug can be substituted.

Lowering of the convulsive threshold is a complication of most neuroleptics. It appears to be dose related, and more of a problem with the low potency phenothiazines. Thus, antipsychotics must be used cautiously in epileptics; and anticonvulsant dosage may need to be increased.

Drug Interactions

The **central sedative effects** of antipsychotics are additive when given with other drugs which have CNS depressant properties. Of particular concern are drugs that can depress respiration (narcotics, barbiturates). The **anticholinergic properties** likewise will be additive to those of other drugs with these effects.

Combinations with **antihypertensives** such as reserpine, alpha-methyl-dopa, or propranolol of those antipsychotics which have alpha-adrenergic blocking properties may have additive effects, resulting in a more pronounced degree of hypotension. Chlorpromazine blocks quanethidine from reaching its receptor site, reversing the antihypertensive effect of quanethidine. The neuroleptics antagonize the effects of levodopa and amphetamine.

The effects of **cardiac drugs** such as quinidine and digitalis may be potentiated by those antipsychotics that prolong ventricular repolarization, increasing the likelihood of a ventricular arrhythmia.

Geltype **antacids** (e.g., Maalox) inhibit oral absorption and decrease serum levels of chlorpromazine and probably other phenothiazines. Antacids should be given either 2 hours before or after chlorpromazine. **Trihexyphenidyl** also lowers serum chlorpromazine levels, presumably by interfering with its absorption. **Barbiturates** lower serum chlorpromazine (and probably other neuroleptics) levels, but by the induction of hepatic microsomal enzymes.

Tricyclic antidepressants inhibit the metabolism of antipsychotic agents, thus leading to higher serum levels of the latter. The reverse also appears to be true. Thus, when given together they potentiate each other, and **both should be given in lower doses** than when administered separately.

Methylphenidate (Ritalin) inhibits the metabolism of phenothiazines and can potentiate their clinical effects. Phenothiazines may potentiate the effects of **oral hypoglycemic agents.**

Antidepressant Agents

The main classes of antidepressant drugs used today are the tricyclic antidepressants and the monoamine oxidase inhibitors (MAOI's). The amphetamines are best thought of as CNS stimulants, not antidepressants, and are of very limited, if any, use in the treatment of depressive illness.

Indications for Use

MAJOR AFFECTIVE (DEPRESSIVE) DISORDERS

These are the primary indication for these drugs. *"Endogenous" depressions (melancholia)* are especially responsive. These are characterized by the presence of biological-vegetative symptoms accompanying the mood disturbance: anorexia, weight loss, insomnia (especially early morning awakening), dry mouth, constipation and psychomotor abnormalities. Often there is diurnal variation in mood, and intense guilt.

Both *unipolar* and *bipolar* depressions respond. In addition, antidepressants may be effective in preventing recurrent unipolar depressions.

Major depressions associated with mood congruent *psychotic features* (primarily delusions) also respond. (Many of these patients would have been diagnosed as *Involutional Melancholia* or as *Psychotic Depressions* in older nomenclature.) Although an antidepressant alone may be effective, the addition of a neuroleptic sometimes is required to ameliorate the psychotic symptoms and agitation.

OTHER AFFECTIVE DISORDERS

Neurotic Depression (Dysthymic disorder) also may respond. This is more likely if some endogenous symptoms (as described above) are present.

Atypical depression is a diagnostic term used for a **specific syndrome** in which there are symptoms of fatigue and somatic complaints accompanied by phobic anxiety. It presents most often as a chronic condition without the classical features of endogenous depression, and is an indication for the use of MAO inhibitors.

SCHIZOAFFECTIVE DISORDERS

The presence of a depressed mood state concomitant with schizophrenic symptoms (see pp. 59–60) may benefit from the addition of an antidepressant to the basic treatment with a neuroleptic. Caution is required, however, for antidepressants sometimes worsen the psychosis.

MISCELLANEOUS USES

Enuresis in children and adolescents may respond to tricyclic antidepressants, although relapse is usual; and there are superior treatments (see Chapter 11). **Chronic pain** may respond to tricyclics. However, the exact mechanism of action is unclear, and may be unrelated to the antidepressant effect. Both the tricyclics and MAOI's are effective in treating the *cataplexy* (extreme muscular weakness) associated with the **narcolepsy** syndrome. Imipramine is the drug of choice, but will not help the core symptom of excessive sleepiness, for which CNS stimulants are required.

Mechanism of Action

There is evidence that depression is associated with relative or absolute deficiency in the amount of available norepinephrine and serotonin at CNS synapses. Both classes of antidepressants increase the concentration of these neurotransmitters; and this is the likely basis for their action. The tricyclics block their reuptake back into the presynaptic neuron. The MAOI's block their intracellular metabolic degradation.

Tricyclic Antidepressants

The tricyclics are rapidly and completely absorbed after oral ingestion. Although some are available in injectable form, IM use does not hasten their onset of action, and may be associated with an increased incidence of cardiovascular side effects. Their plasma half-life is approximately 24 hours or longer. Thus, they can be administered on a once-a-day basis.

There may be a tenfold difference in plasma levels in patients receiving the same dosage of drug. Thus, **dose regimens must be highly individualized.** At present, it is difficult to specify the optimal plasma level of any tricyclic. However, studies with nortriptyline have suggested an effective therapeutic range to be 50 to 150 ng/ml. Levels below or above this have been associated with poor clinical response: a pattern referred to as the "therapeutic window." The correlation between serum levels and clinical response for other tricyclics has generally been linear: the higher the serum level, the better the response.

A key feature of the tricyclics is the **delay in the onset of their clinical action.** Although some patients may show significant improvement in 1 week, 2 to 4 weeks at therapeutic doses is generally required before the maximal antidepressant effect is seen.

The tricyclics have varying degrees of sedative effects. They also have potent central and peripheral anticholinergic effects. In general, the more sedating a tricyclic, the more potent are its anticholinergic effects.

The tricyclic antidepressants currently available in this country are listed in Table 3 with their trade and generic names, and usual dose ranges.

Amitriptyline is the **most anticholinergic,** and along with doxepin, also the **most sedative.** It is especially useful for those depressions in which anxiety or agitation and insomnia are prominent symptoms. Its strong anticholinergic side effects are often tolerated poorly by the elderly, who may develop a toxic delirium similar to atropine toxicity. (This is manifested by disorientation, confusion, agitation, recent memory loss, and visual hallucinations.)

Table 3. Approximate Daily Dose Ranges of Antidepressant Drugs[a]

Generic Name	Trade Name	Usual Daily Dose Range (mg/day)	
		Inpatient	Outpatient or Maintenance
Tricyclic antidepressants			
Tertiary amines			
Amitriptyline	Elavil, Endep	150–300	50–150
Doxcpin	Sinequan, Adapin	150–300	50–150
Imipramine	Tofranil, Presamine	150–300	50–150
Trimipramine	Surmontil	150–300	50–150
Secondary amines			
Desipramine	Norpramin, Pertofrane	150–300	50–150
Nortriptyline	Aventyl, Pamelor	75–200	25–100
Protriptyline	Vivactil	30–60	10–30
Amoxapine	Asendin	200–300[b]	150–300[c]
Monoamine oxidase inhibitors			
Phenelzine	Nardil	45–75	15–45
Tranylcypromine	Parnate	20–30	10–20

[a]*Note:* Amitriptyline and imipramine are also available generically.
[b]May be cautiously raised up to 600 mg/day if no response after 2 weeks.
[c]May be cautiously raised up to 400 mg/day if no response after 2 weeks.

Nortriptyline is the demethylated metabolite of amitriptyline and more potent on a weight basis. It is less sedative and less anticholinergic than most tricyclics.

Imipramine is intermediate in its sedative and anticholinergic effects. As the first marketed tricyclic, its effectiveness in depression has been well established; and it has been used more extensively for other indications than the others.

Desipramine is the demethylated metabolite of imipramine. It is the **least anticholinergic** and therefore useful for patients in whom such side effects might prove troublesome (e.g., the elderly, those with prostatic hypertrophy or glaucoma). It is the second least sedating.

Doxepin, along with amitriptyline, is **strongly sedating.** After amitriptyline it is the second most **anticholinergic.** It is the weakest inhibitor of neurotransmitter reuptake and, therefore, the least potent drug of this class. Its main advantage is that it appears to have the fewest cardiovascular side effects, and thus may be particularly useful in those patients with cardiac problems.

Protriptyline is the **least sedating and may in fact be stimulating.** Thus, it may be especially useful in withdrawn or retarded depressions. It is the most potent tricyclic on a mg/mg basis and has the **longest action** (half-life of 54 to 198 hours). Clinically, its anticholinergic effects appear to be intermediate.

Imipramine, amitriptyline, and doxepin are tertiary amines, while desipramine, nortriptyline, and protriptyline are secondary amines. In general, the secondary amines are less sedating and have less anticholinergic effects than the tertiary amines. The secondary amines preferentially block the reuptake of norepinephrine, while the tertiary amines are more potent blockers of serotonin reuptake.

Recently Marketed Antidepressants

Maprotiline (Ludiomil) is the first *tetracyclic* antidepressant available in this country. It has been shown to be as effective as the tricyclics and MAOI's in the treatment of depression, but appears to produce fewer and less severe cardiovascular and anticholinergic side effects than the tricyclics.

Trimipramine (Surmontil), a new tricyclic, appears to be as efficacious as imipramine and amitriptyline in several controlled studies; and has a similar dose range. It is similar to imipramine structurally, but is more sedating. Its other side effects are anticholinergic actions and postural hypotension.

Amoxapine (Asendin), the newest tricyclic, equals imipramine and amitriptyline in efficacy. It has often been shown to have a significantly **earlier onset of action** than other tricyclics: as little as 4 to 7 days. Its dose range is 50 to 600 mg/day, with most patients responding to 200 to 300 mg. The most commonly observed side effects are sedation and anticholinergic effects; but cardiotoxic effects appear to be infrequent.

Trazodone (Desyrel), while at the time of writing not yet approved for use in the United States, is expected to be approved soon. This drug represents an entirely different class of antidepressant than the tricyclics and MAO inhibitors. It appears to be a selective inhibitor of serotonin reuptake; and is reported to have antianxiety effects in addition to antidepressant activity. Trazodone has been found to be equal in efficacy to the tricyclics, and has a similarly delayed onset of action. Of significance is the fact that it produces **minimal cardiovascular and anticholinergic side effects.** Other side effects are reported to be mild. (Most commonly reported are drowsiness, dizziness, headache, lethargy, GI distress, and insomnia.) Dose schedules resemble those for the tricyclics.

Limbitrol is a combination of a tricyclic antidepressant (amitriptyline) and a benzodiazepine (chlordiazepoxide). Marketed for depression accompanied by significant anxiety, it may also be useful for patients who experience overstimulation, restlessness, jitteriness, or insomnia on a tricyclic alone. The advantage of this combination over that with a neuroleptic (e.g., amitriptyline and perphenazine) is that there is no risk of developing tardive dyskinesia. All combinations are inflexible, so that the drugs should be used separately, at least initially, to establish the correct dosage of each.

Monoamine Oxidase Inhibitors (MAOI's)

Phenelzine and *tranylcypromine* are the two most commonly used drugs of this class. These drugs have minimal, if any, sedative or anticholinergic effects. They may produce unwanted stimulation, especially tranylcypromine. Both drugs produce long-lasting MAO inhibition, and therefore can be administered once a day. Phenelzine is similar to the tricyclics in that it generally takes 2 to 3 weeks before its full antidepressant effect is seen. Tranylcypromine is quicker acting, reportedly in approximately 10 days. Tranylcypromine is also more potent, and probably more effective. However, the risk of serious side effects, particularly hypertensive crises, is also greater with its use.

These compounds are extremely tricky to use because of **potentially serious side effects.** Thus, they are not the antidepressants of choice (except in atypical depressions) but are used only if the tricyclics fail or are contraindicated. Consequently, other than in very rare instances **their prescription should be limited to psychiatrists** familiar with their use.

Hypertensive crises have occurred when patients taking MAOI's have ingested foods containing tyramine or medications containing sympathomimetic agents. Although these reactions are rare, the are potentially fatal. **Patients taking MAOI's must avoid tyramine-containing foods:** aged cheeses, beer and wine, broadbean pods (fava beans), pickled herring, canned figs, sour cream, chicken livers, and yeast extracts (e.g., Bovril and Marmite). Caffeine-containing beverages and chocolate should be used only in moderation because of their sympathomimetic effects. Medications containing decongestants (cold and sinus medications), amphetamines or levodopa, which are sympathomimetic amines, must be avoided, as must reserpine.

Guidelines for Clinical Use

TRICYCLIC ANTIDEPRESSANTS

The selection of a tricyclic for any given patient is based on clinical grounds. (Pharmacologic studies hold promise of laboratory predictors, but have not achieved clinical usefulness.) A personal or family drug response history may be useful. **Generally, one bases choice on the degree of sedative and anticholinergic properties** of each of the tricyclics. For example, amitriptyline would be appropriate for a depressed patient with anxiety and insommia; desipramine for one in whom anticholinergic side effects could be troublesome; and protriptyline for one with lethargy and psychomotor retardation. In a patient with cardiac problems, doxepin could be used.

Treatment should be initiated with low, divided doses (e.g., imipramine at 25 mg t.i.d.). If well tolerated, the dose should be increased gradually to about midway in the effective range (see Table 3). If well tolerated, the drug can be **gradually shifted to a single bedtime dose;** or two-thirds of the total can be given then. This may provide sedation for sleep, and decrease daytime side effects. Doses for elderly patients should be approximately one-third to one-half of those for younger adults, increased more gradually, and kept on a divided schedule. Similar precautions should be taken for patients with cardiovascular problems.

The patient should be left on the selected dosage for approximately 2 weeks, and then evaluated for signs of improvement. If improvement is satisfactory, that dose can be maintained. If no definite sign of improvement are apparent, and presuming the drug is well tolerated, the dose should be gradually increased by 25 mg every few days to the top of the range listed in Table 3. In general, the dose can be increased until improvement is noted or troublesome side effects intervene.

The most common errors are using too low a dose and not giving tricyclics for a long enough period to be effective. The therapeutic effect may not even begin until 10 to 14 days after an effective dose has been reached.

After maximal dosage has been reached, 4 to 6 weeks on that regimen is an adequate trial. If improvement is not optimal by then, the patient should be considered refractory, and another treatment instituted. If a patient is refractory to a tertiary amine, one could shift to a secondary amine which would exert its major effect on a different neurotransmitter (e.g., from amitriptyline to desipramine). If a patient has been refractory to two tricyclics, it would seem prudent to try a MAOI or electrocon-vulsive therapy (ECT). (The use of ECT is described in Chapter 7.)

Maintenance treatment is considered after optimal response is achieved. It is probably best to leave the patient on the therapeutic dose for 6 to 8 weeks. After this, it may be tapered by 25 mg every 1 to 2 weeks until an effective maintenance level is reached: often about one-half the therapeutic dose, although there is considerable variation. If any signs of relapse occur, one should reinstitute the last previously effective dose. After 6 to 8 weeks on this dose, tapering may be tried again.

Generally, maintenance treatment should be continued for 6 to 8 months during which the patient has been symptom-free, although patients with mild first depressive episodes may be discontinued earlier. Some patients may require prolonged maintenance therapy, while those with frequent recurrent depressions may need maintenance treatment indefinitely. In either case, the lowest effective dose should be used. This may be very low—well below that necessary for treatment.

The tricyclics can be fatal if an overdose is taken (10 times the therapeutic dose can be lethal), unlike the neuroleptics which have a wide margin of safety. Because many depressed patients are suicide prone, often **it is best not to prescribe more than a one week's supply** of medication at a time.

MAO INHIBITORS
Most of the guidelines for the use of tricyclics also apply to the MAOI's. However, there are some differences. The starting doses for phenelzine and tranylcypromine are also often effective therapeutic doses. Any increase in dose should be gradual. An adequate clinical trial of phenelzine is 60 to 75 mg/day for 4 weeks, while that for tranylcypromine is 30 mg/day for 2 weeks. Single daily doses of MAOI's are best given in the morning, as bedtime doses may cause unwanted stimulation. Maintenance regimens for MAOI's have not been as well established as those for tricyclics. **Like the tricyclics, MAOI's have a narrow margin of safety;** and an overdose can be fatal. The same prescribing precautions apply.

The combination of a tricyclic and a MAOI has been reported to cause dangerous side effects. There should be a 7- to 14-day **washout period** of a drug of one class before starting the other. (The cautious combination of a tricyclic and a MAOI has been reported efficacious in refractory depressions; but its use should be left to the expert.)

Side Effects

TRICYCLIC ANTIDEPRESSANTS

Anticholinergic effects are as described under the antipsychotics. Bethanecol (Urecholine) in doses up to 75 mg/day has been found to be useful in counteracting these. Tricyclics should be prescribed with caution in patients with glaucoma or prostatic hypertrophy. A toxic confusional state may occur in the elderly, or with overdoses. This is treated with physostigmine (Antilirium) 1 to 2 mg IM (or slowly IV), repeated at 30- to 45-minute intervals until symptoms clear permanently.

Cardiovascular effects include **postural hypotension, tachycardia, and palpitations.** The tricyclics also have a **quinidine-like action** and can produce changes in cardiac conduction. The EKG may show prolongation of the P-R and Q-T intervals, depression of the S-T segment, flattening of the T-wave and, more rarely, bundle branch block. Arrhythmias (both supraventricular and ventricular) may occur, particularly following an overdose. As with the phenothiazines, prolongation of cardiac repolarization increases the chances of developing a reentry arrhythmia. Direct suppression of the myocardium and precipitation of congestive heart failure have been reported. Patients with a history of cardiac disease are at greater risk; and tricyclics must be used with caution in this population.

CNS effects include **excessive sedation,** which can be diminished by using a single bedtime dose. Tricyclics can produce a fine resting **tremor** which may be controlled with either diazepam or propranolol. **Restlessness, insomnia, and agitation** may occur. hould this happen, switching to another tricyclic may prove helpful. The combination of amitriptyline and perphenazine may be useful for patients who have these symptoms on tricyclics alone. Like the antipsychotics, tricyclics **lower the convulsive threshold** and may cause seizures in susceptible patients, although not commonly. Anticonvulsant dosage may need to be adjusted in epileptic patients.

Manic episodes may be precipitated. Patients with bipolar affective disorders, especially, may move directly into a manic state following relief of the depression.

Schizophrenic attacks also may be precipitated, especially in patients with a schizoid or borderline personality disorder, or a history of schizophrenia. The combination of a neuroleptic and a tricyclic may be useful in such patients.

Other side effects include weight gain, which may be due, in part, to improvement of the depression. Allergic skin reactions and excessive sweating may occur. Cholestatic jaundice, purpura, eosinophilia, and agranulocytosis are rare.

MAO INHIBITORS

Orthostatic(postural) hypotension is common.

CNS effects include agitation, restlessness, insomnia, anxiety, and irritability.

Manic or psychotic episodes may be precipitated, as with tricyclics.

Hypertensive crisis. **This can be very dangerous, although it is rare with proper diet control** (see p. 236). The treatment of choice is phentolamine (Regitine) given slowly IV.

Other side effects include skin rashes, constipation, dry mouth, headache, weakness, and impotence. Leukopenia has been reported occasionally with phenelzine. Hepatotoxicity may rarely occur.

Drug Interactions

TRICYCLIC ANTIDEPRESSANTS

The central sedative effects of the tricyclics are additive when given with other drugs that have CNS-depressant properties (e.g., alcohol, sedative–hypnotics). **The anticholinergic properties** of the tricyclics will also be additive to those of other drugs with these effects (e.g., antiparkinsonian drugs). **The cardiotoxic effects** of the tricyclics are additive with those of thioridazine and with quinidine.

Tricyclics block the action of **guanethidine** (Ismelin) and **clonidine** (Catapres), and thus reverse the hypotensive effects of these drugs. The exception is doxepin in low doses (150 mg/day or less).

Barbiturates increase the metabolism of tricyclics through the induction of hepatic enzymes. Thus they decrease serum tricyclic levels. Chloral hydrate has been reported to have a similar effect. **Phenothiazines, butyrophenones, and methylphenidate** (Ritalin), in contrast, retard the metabolism of tricyclics and thus increase their serum levels.

Dicumarol action may be prolonged by nortriptyline. Interference with the absorption of **levodopa and phenylbutazone** has been reported with tricyclics. The hypertensive and arrhythmia producing effects of **sympathomimetic amines** can be potentiated.

MAO INHIBITORS

The effects of CNS depressants, insulin, and oral hypoglycemic agents are potentiated. Other drugs potentiated by MAOI's include amphetamines, anticholinergics, hypotensive diuretics, and smooth muscle relaxants.

The combination of a MAOI and meperidine (Demerol) has been associated with hyperpyrexia, seizures, extreme excitement, and reactions like a narcotic overdose. **The use of a narcotic in a patient taking a MAOI should be avoided.**

Lithium

Lithium should be prescribed **only** by physicians who are thoroughly familiar with its use.

Indications for Use

Lithium is indicated for **the treatment of mania and for the prevention of recurrences of bipolar manic–depressive illness.** (It may be effective in the prevention of recurrences of unipolar manic–depressive illness, but is not yet approved for this use.) Although lithium cannot be considered a standard drug for the treatment of depression, it may be efficacious for bipolar depressed patients, or those patients refractory to all other treatments.

Chemical and Pharmacologic Properties

Lithium is the lightest known metal, belonging to the same group as sodium and potassium. *Lithium carbonate* is the salt used for therapeutic purposes. It is rapidly absorbed from the GI tract, reaching peak plasma levels in 30 minutes to 2 hours. There is no evidence of protein binding; nor is it metabolized. These features allow serum lithium levels to be easily and accurately measured in the laboratory.

The plasma half-life is approximately 24 hours, and steady-state concentrations are reached in about 5 days. Lithium is almost completely excreted by the kidneys, and the rate of lithium excretion varies directly with serum sodium levels. High sodium intake increases lithium excretion, while low sodium intake decreases lithium excretion and thus raises serum lithium levels. This relationship is important because **patients on diuretics or low-salt diets can develop lithium toxicity,** if not monitored closely.

Guidelines for Clinical Use

Pretreatment workup. In addition to a thorough medical history and physical examination, the following baseline laboratory studies should be done prior to treatment:

Renal function studies: urinalysis, blood urea nitrogen (BUN), serum creatinine, and 24-hour urine for total volume and creatinine clearance.

Thyroid function studies: serum T_3 and T_4 levels.

Electrolytes: serum sodium and potassium levels.

Complete blood count: since lithium can cause a reversible leukocytosis, it is advisable to obtain a baseline white blood cell count.

Electrocardiogram: an EKG should be obtained if there is any suspicion of cardiovascular disease or risk of developing cardiovascular problems. (Renal or cardiac disease requiring the use of diuretics or salt restriction are relative contraindications to lithium use.)

Treatment with lithium is monitored with blood levels. Levels should be **drawn 10 to 12 hours after the last dose.** All recommended therapeutic levels are based on this interval.

Lithium is generally given in divided doses, two to four times per day. This tends to decrease the incidence of side effects. GI side effects can be further diminished by giving lithium after meals. Lithium carbonate is available in 300-mg capsules and tablets; although both are equally efficacious, some patients report more GI distress with the tablets.

Treatment of Mania

Acute manic episodes are best treated in the hospital. The initial dose is generally 600 to 900 mg/day. This is increased gradually until a serum lithium level between **1.0 and 1.5 mEq/L** is reached, the effective range for treatment of acute mania. If an initial dose is well tolerated, this can be doubled the second day. The serum level should be determined every 3 to 4 days during the early stages of treatment, and the dosage adjusted accordingly until a therapeutic level is reached. After the patient becomes stabilized on a given dose, serum levels can be checked weekly.

Lithium's **slow onset of action** (7 to 10 days) often makes it necessary to use an antipsychotic agent simultaneously during the early stage of treatment. After the lithium becomes effective, the antipsychotic can be tapered and discontinued.

After significant remission has occurred, the lithium dose can be decreased to a maintenance level. Otherwise, a patient should receive maximally tolerated doses (up to a serum level of 1.5 mEq/L) for a period of 3 weeks. If he does not respond in that time, he should be considered refractory to lithium and another treatment (e.g., an antipsychotic agent) instituted.

Maintenance Treatment (Prophylaxis)

Patients with one or more episodes of manic–depressive disorder per year should be considered for maintenance therapy. Maintenance is often a continuation of the treatment of an acute episode, but may be initiated while the patient is in remission. The serum lithium range for maintenance treatment is **0.6 to 1.2 mEq/L.** (Some clinicians prefer 0.5 to 1.0 to reduce the risk of side effects.) If a patient is to be started directly on maintenance therapy, lithium can be initiated at 600 to 900 mg/day, a serum level drawn in 1 week, and the dose adjusted accordingly. Serum levels then should be drawn weekly until the level is consistently in the therapeutic range. Once a patient is stabilized on a given dose, levels need only be drawn every 4 to 6 weeks. Patients who have been on the drug for long periods of time may have blood levels drawn even less frequently. **Renal function should be reevaluated every 6 months, and thyroid function reevaluated annually.**

Side Effects

Side effects may occur at serum levels about 1.0 mEq/L, and are more common at levels of about 1.5. However, they may be seen at lower levels.

Gastrointestinal symptoms are common during the early weeks of treatment. They include anorexia, nausea, and loose stools. These are often mild and diminish with continued treatment. Less frequently, vomiting, abdominal pains, and diarrhea may occur. **Reappearance of GI symptoms may be the first indicator of toxicity.**

Neurological side effects are also fairly common during the early phases of treatment. These include fatigue, muscle weakness, a dazed feeling, malaise, and a fine tremor of the hands. The tremor may persist, but often can be controlled with propranolol (Inderal) in doses of 20 to 60 mg/day.

Renal. Mild polyuria and polydipsia are fairly common during the early weeks of treatment. More rarely, a reversible form of nephrogenic diabetes insipidus may occur, associated with marked polyuria and polydipsia. This may necessitate discontinuation of treatment, if it does not respond to a reduction in dose. Recent studies have shown changes in both renal function and pathology in patients who have been on chronic lithium maintenance. The most common findings have been a decrease in renal concentrating ability, a decreased creatinine clearance, focal nephron atrophy, and interstitial fibrosis.

Cardiac. EKG changes similar to those seen with hypokalemia (flattening and inversion of the T-wave) may occur. These are benign and reversible. Rarely, PVCs and sinus node arrhythmias may occur.

Thyroid. Hypothyroidism, with or without the development of goiter, may be seen. This is 10 times more common in women. **Hypothyroidism must be distinguished from depression.** A nontoxic goiter with normal thyroid function also may occur. Patients with an underlying thyroid defect appear to be at greater risk. These effects are more common with chronic lithium use, but may occur after several weeks of treatment. Hypothyroidism is reversible upon stopping lithium, but is easily treated by administering thyroxin and does not require discontinuation of the drug. The same is generally true for goiter.

Leukocytosis has been observed, with WBC counts up to 14,000 to 15,000/mm³. It appears to be benign, and is reversible upon discontinuation of lithium.

Teratogencity. There appears to be a higher incidence of cardiovascular malformations in babies born to mothers who received lithium during the first trimester of pregnancy. Lithium should be avoided during pregnancy, especially the first trimester.

Other side effects reported include weight gain, edema, altered carbohydrate metabolism, exophthalmos, hypercalcemia, and a variety of skin disorders.

Lithium Toxicity

Toxicity generally occurs at serum levels above 2.0 mEq/L, but may occur at therapeutic levels in predisposed individuals. Elderly patients, patients with preexisting organic brain syndrome, and schizophrenics appear to be at greater risk. Toxicity occurring at therapeutic doses may be due to impaired renal function, the use of diuretics, salt restriction, or dehydration (secondary to vomiting, diarrhea, heat stroke, or fever).

Lithium toxicity does not occur abruptly. Warning signs may be present for several days. **Early signs of toxicity may include nausea, vomiting, and diarrhea.**

However, **it is the central nervous system that is primarily involved in lithium toxicity.** Early CNS signs of toxicity may include sluggishness, drowsiness, dysarthria, blurred vision, ataxia, a coarse tremor, and muscle twitching or fasciculation. As toxicity progresses, one may see confusion, decreasing levels of consciousness, nystagmus, myoclonic movements, hyperactive deep tendon reflexes, a Babinski response, choreoathetoid movements, increased muscle tonus, incontinence, and seizures. If untreated, **lithium toxicity can lead to permanent neurologic damage or coma and death.** Dementia, choreoathetoid movements, and cerebellar signs have been reported.

The treatment of lithium toxicity consists of discontinuation of the drug, proper attention to electrolyte balance, and general supportive measures. In severe intoxication, hemodialysis may be required.

Drug Interactions

Most **diuretics** cause lithium retention, and increase serum levels. Drugs that increase lithium excretion, and therefore decrease serum lithium levels, include: osmotic diuretics (e.g., mannitol); acetazolamide; xanthine derivatives (e.g., aminophylline); and sodium bicarbonate.

Lowered chlorpromazine levels have been reported due to lithium. **Prolonged activity of neuromuscular blocking drugs** can occur. Since succinylcholine is commonly used during ECT, lithium should be discontinued prior to ECT.

Lithium can be safely and efficaciously used with either the tricyclic antidepressants or MAO inhibitors (or neuroleptics). There is some evidence that the combination of lithium and a tricyclic antidepressant has a synergistic effect.

Benzodiazepines

The **benzodiazepines are the drugs of choice in the treatment of anxiety and insomnia.** This newer class of drugs, also called anxiolytics or minor tranquilizers, has proven to be more effective and safer than all prior agents for these problems, making the older agents almost obsolete.

Indications for Use

ANXIETY OF A NONPSYCHOTIC NATURE

This is their principal indication. These drugs are **most useful in anxiety that is severe and acute,** reactive to environmental or internal stress, and accompanied by physical tension, agitation, or apprehension. Anticipatory anxiety (e.g., prior to surgery) also responds well. Anxiety that is short-lived or transient responds better; **chronic, neurotic anxiety responds poorly** and is best treated with psychotherapy. If medication is necessary in treating chronic anxiety, it should be used only at times of maximal stress. In general, medication should not be prescribed unless anxiety is severe enough to interfere with the patient's activities of daily living (e.g., work, interpersonal relationships). Even when the benzodiazepines are used, they should be thought of as adjuncts to psychotherapy, which will help provide more effective, permanent ways of coping with stress and anxiety.

INSOMNIA

Whenever possible, **the primary disorder responsible should be treated** (e.g. hypothyroidism, depression). If hypnotic drugs are indicated, their use should be occasional and in the lowest possible doses. Of all the agents presently used as hypnotics, the benzodiazepines appear to interfere least with normal physiologic sleep, including rapid eye movement (REM) stage sleep. Although flurazepam is widely promoted for insomnia, other benzodiazepines may be equally efficacious.

ALCOHOL WITHDRAWAL

The benzodiazepines have become **the treatment of choice** for the alcohol withdrawal syndrome. They are cross-tolerant with alcohol, have a wider margin of safety than the barbiturates and paraldehyde, and do not lower the convulsive threshold as do the antipsychotics.

ACUTE PSYCHOSES SECONDARY TO HALLUCINOGENIC DRUGS

Such reactions to LSD etc. are an indication for the benzodiazepines, if pharmacologic intervention is necessary. Simple "talking-down" may suffice. **The antipsychotics are generally contraindicated** in such cases because they may potentiate the anticholinergic effects of belladonna alkaloids which are often covertly included in illicit preparations.

MUSCLE SPASM

The benzodiazepines, particularly diazepam, have muscle-relaxing effects useful in treating spasm (e.g., back strain, neurological disorders). Thus, they are doubly useful in anxiety-induced muscle tension.

PSYCHOPHYSIOLOGICAL DISORDERS

These agents are much overused in these conditions as substitutes for effective general psychotherapeutic management. They may be useful as adjuncts, however, if somatic symptoms arise from actual physiological changes associated with emotional arousal.

NONPSYCHIATRIC USES

They have important value as **anticonvulsants,** especially in status epilepticus. Various benzodiazepines have use also for preoperative medication and for brief anaesthesia.

Chemical and Pharmacologic Properties

The benzodiazepines have several advantages over the other classes of antianxiety and hyponotic agents. They have a **wide therapeutic range,** having antianxiety effects in low doses, and hypnotic effects in higher doses. Relief of anxiety can be obtained with little production of sedation or drowsiness. They have a **wide margin of safety,** and overdose is rarely lethal when taken alone. They do not interfere with the metabolism of other drugs which may be taken concurrently. In contrast to the barbiturates and meprobamate, tolerance develops slowly. Although physiological addiction can occur, it generally involves the use of high doses over several months' time. **The biggest problem is habituation or psychological dependence.** Physicians have contributed to this by overprescribing. Paradoxically, the low acute toxicity contributes to this, producing a false sense of security. Another factor in overprescribing is misuse as a placebo in place of needed psychotherapeutic management. Due to their longer duration of action, withdrawal syndromes following prolonged use are less severe than those of barbiturates or meprobamate.

A list of the available benzodiazepines is provided in Table 4, which includes trade and generic names, usual dose range and duration of action.

Chlordiazepoxide is the oldest of the benzodiazepines. It is available generically, and is the least expensive. It is promptly absorbed after oral ingestion, reaching peak plasma levels in 1 to 4 hours. IM absorption is erratic, and serum levels have been shown to be higher after oral administration; thus, IM use is avoided. It may be given IV, if parenteral administration is required. The plasma half-life ranges from 6 to 30 hours; however, it is transformed into three active metabolites which prolong its activity. One of these (desmethyldiazepam) is very long-acting (half-life: 48 to 96 hours). Thus, chlordiazepoxide has **a tendency to accumulate** when given several times a day. This is more likely in the elderly, and patients with impaired liver function, who metabolize the drug more slowly. Heavy smokers appear to metabolize this drug more rapidly.

Diazepam is highly lipid soluble and water insoluble, in contrast to water-soluble chlordiazepoxide. Parenteral preparations will precipitate

Table 4. The Benzodiazepines

Generic Name	Trade Name	Usual Daily Dose Range[a] (mg/day)	Duration of Action
Antianxiety agents			
Chlordiazepoxide[b]	Librium[c]	15–100	Long
Clorazepate dipotassium	Tranxene	15–60	Long
Clorazepate monopotassium	Azene	13–52	Long
Diazepam[b]	Valium	6–40	Long
Lorazepam[b]	Ativan	1–6	Intermediate
Oxazepam	Serax	30–120	Short
Prazepam	Centrax	20–60	Long
Hypnotic–sedatives			
Flurazepam	Dalmane	15–30 (at	Long
Temazepam	Restoril	15–30 bedtime)	Short

[a]Higher doses may be needed for the treatment of alcohol withdrawal.
[b]Available in parenteral form.
[c]Chlordrazepoxide is also available generically.

if diluted with water or saline. It is rapidly absorbed from the GI tract, but, like chlordiazepoxide, erratically and incompletely absorbed after IM administration. It can be used IV, but slowly—to avoid respiratory depression. Its plasma half-life is 20 to 50 hours, but it is metabolized even more slowly by the elderly. It also has three active metabolites, one of which is desmethyldiazepam. Another is oxazepam (see below). Hence, **diazepam will accumulate** if doses are given too frequently. Recently, diazepam has become popular as **a drug of abuse.** Its rapid absorption and high potency can combine to produce acute intoxication.

Oxazepam, a metabolite of diazepam, has no active metabolites of its own and has the shortest half-life of any benzodiazepine (approximately 7 hours). Thus there is little tendency for it to accumulate; and may be **particularly useful in the elderly or in patients with impaired liver function.** It is reported to be the most potent anticonvulsant of the benzodiazepines, and may be particularly suited for alcohol withdrawal. Oxazepam is well absorbed orally, although not as rapidly as diazepam. Peak plasma levels are reached in 2 to 4 hours.

Lorazepam is one of the newer benzodiazepines. It is well absorbed orally, and peak plasma levels are reached 2 hours after ingestion. Its plasma half-life is 12 to 15 hours. Like oxazepam it has no active metabolites, and has less tendency to accumulate.

Clorazepate, though not an active substance itself, is converted to desmethyldiazepam which has prolonged activity. Normal gastric acidity is required for this; thus, **antacids or achlorhydria interfere with its efficacy. Accumulation can become a problem.** Clorazepate is marketed as the dipotassium salt (Tranxene) and the monopotassium salt (Azene).

Prazepam is a more recently marketed benzodiazepine. Absorbed slowly after oral administration, its clinical activity is due mainly to its major active metabolite, desmethyldiazepam. The latter reaches peak plasma levels in about 6 hours; and its half-life is approximately 48–96 hours; so that accumulation can occur.

Flurazepam has been promoted for its hypnotic effects. There is a smaller margin between the dose required for antianxiety effects and that to induce sleep. It is effective for both sleep induction and maintenance. It is well absorbed orally. Hypnotic effects are generally seen within an hour, and last for 7 to 8 hours. It has been shown to be effective for up to 28 days of consecutive use. It has a very short half-life, but its major metabolite has a very long one (47 to 100 hours). Thus, **accumulation** of this metabolite can occur after repeated doses, especially in the elderly or those with liver disorders. Clinically, drug hangover is not a frequent problem.

Temazepam, the newest available benzodiazepine, also is marketed for its hypnotic effects. Its half-life is reported to be approximately 10 hours; and it has no active metabolites. Hence is has much less tendency to accumulate.

Guidelines for Clinical Use

ANXIETY

Since all of the benzodiazepines are efficacious, **the choice of a particular drug should be made on the basis of its pharmacokinetic properties.** For example, oxazepam and lorazepam may be especially useful when drug accumulation is undesirable. Steady-state conditions of these drugs are reached at approximately five times the half-life.

Oxazepam is usually prescribed three to four times per day because of its short half-life; Lorazepam two to three times per day. The other benzodiazepines may be initially prescribed two to three times per day until a steady state is reached. The schedule can then be shifted to once or twice a day. Using smaller daily doses initially helps avoid accumulation. Prescribing all or the majority of the longer-acting drugs at bedtime may aid sleep and avoid excessive daytime sedation.

Once a patient is started on a benzodiazepine, he should be followed every 1 to 2 weeks. Changes in the nature of the anxiety warrant changes in the dose. At all times, the lowest possible dose should be used. Dose ranges are listed in Table 4.

The duration of use depends on individual patient requirements. Since anxiety is frequently episodic, **short courses** (a few weeks or less) should be the rule rather than the exception. Long term treatment runs the **risk of tolerance and habituation.**

As improvement is noted, the dosage should be gradually reduced and discontinued, not abruptly stopped, in order to avoid withdrawal symptoms. Some patients find it reassuring to take the medication on a p.r.n. basis for a **brief** time before discontinuation.

INSOMNIA

Flurazepam is currently the drug of choice. It is generally prescribed in a 30-mg dose at bedtime. Elderly patients or those with liver dysfunction should be given 15 mg. Its use should be confined to short periods. It has not been shown to be effective for longer than 28 consecutive nights.

Sleep laboratory studies have shown that the **chronic use of hypnotics is associated with an impaired sleep pattern.** About 20% of cases of insomnia are caused by hypnotic drug dependency, and can be treated by gradual withdrawal of the drug. Tolerance and habituation are also problems with chronic use.

Side Effects

The main side effects result from **CNS depression.** Drowsiness or oversedation is most common. Poor coordination, ataxia, dysarthria, and confusion may also occur. **Patients should be cautioned about driving,** operating heavy machinery, and using alcohol. Respiratory depression may occur in patients with preexisting respiratory disease. These agents should not be used in patients with respiratory failure. Occasional patients report feeling irritable, angry, or agitated after taking benzodiazepines. More rarely, rage reactions have been reported. These may be due to the disinhibiting effects of these drugs, similar to that seen with alcohol. Other side effects reported include GI discomfort, vertigo, decreased libido, and allergic skin reactions.

Drug Interactions

The **sedative effects** of the benzodiazepines are potentiated by other drugs that have CNS depressant effects.

In addition to interfering with the conversion of clorazepate to desmethyldiazepam, **antacids** have also been reported to delay the absorption of the other benzodiazepines. **Disulfiram** (Antabuse) and **Cimetidine** (Tagamet) have been reported to interfere with the metabolism of chlordiazepoxide and diazepam, but not those benzodiazepines that do not undergo demethylation, such as oxazepam or lorazepam.

The benzodiazepines may potentiate the effects of **phenytoin** (Dilantin), leading to signs of toxicity in some patients. Impaired coordination, ataxia, drowsiness, restlessness, and irritability may result.

Other Hypnotics, Sedatives, and Antianxiety Agents

Barbiturates

Several problems with the barbiturates have led to a deserved decline in their use as antianxiety and hypnotic agents. This use should be rare or nonexistent. They have a **narrow margin of saftey,** the lethal dose being close to the therapeutic dose, because of their pronounced depression of respiratory centers. **Tolerance and addiction** are not uncommon; and **withdrawal** can be serious and life threatening. Barbiturates also induce hepatic enzyme activity, lowering the levels of some other drugs. This interaction with coumarin anticoagulants can lead to a sharp rise in levels upon discontinuation of the barbiturates, resulting in bleeding. Suppression of REM sleep is another unwanted characteristic. REM rebound upon their cessation is often associated with vivid nightmares. The shorter-acting barbiturates (e.g., secobarbital) continue to be **major drugs of abuse.** Barbiturates are the drugs most often **used in successful suicide attempts.** Finally, it is difficult to achieve an adequate antianxiety effect without producing oversedation.

Phenobarbital should not be used for the treatment of anxiety, though it often is. If the barbiturates are used at all as hypnotics, their use should not exceed 2 to 3 days. They may produce paradoxical excitement, especially in the elderly, and may also precipitate or exacerbate acute intermittent porphyria.

Propanediols

Meprobamate and tybamate are representative drugs of this class. They are **no more effective than the barbiturates, and have many of the same problems** (e.g., tolerance, abuse, addiction, withdrawal, and lethality). Addiction can occur at doses not much higher than the upper limit of the therapeutic range.

Chloral Derivatives

Chloral hydrate is the principal drug of this class. It is a **relatively safe hypnotic,** which appears to be better for sleep induction than sleep maintenance. Some clinicians prefer this drug for children and the elderly. However, it tends to lose its effectiveness after several days of use. It does not depress REM sleep or induce hepatic enzyme activity as much as the barbiturates, and it is much less abused. Its main side effect is gastric irritation. It has been reported to potentiate the effects of some drugs by displacing them from protein binding sites.

Sedative Antihistamines

These agents include hydroxyzine (Vistaril, Atarax) and diphenhydramine (Benadryl). Unlike the other sedative hypnotics, they have no muscle relaxing properties and lower the convulsive threshold. They have a low abuse potential, as they produce a mental clouding along with their sedative effect, which patients often find unpleasant. Thus, **diphenhydramine may be a useful short-term hypnotic for patients who have a tendency to abuse drugs.** Many clinicians prefer this as their second choice after flurazepam. These drugs may have a special usefulness in psychophysiologic skin disorders because of their combined sedative and antihistaminic properties. They do have **undesirable anticholinergic side effects;** and tolerance may develop to their sedative effects. Diphenhydramine has been shown to significantly depress REM sleep.

Nonbarbiturate Hypnotics

The use of these drugs is not recommended. They include glutethimide (Doriden), ethchlorvynol (Placidyl), methyprylon (Noludar), and methaqualone (Quaalude and others). In general, they have no advantages over the barbiturates and possess many of the same problems. Gluteth-imide is an extremely lethal drug when taken in overdose. Like the barbiturates it induces hepatic microsomal enzymes and thus decreases the serum levels of other drugs. **Methaqualone is a popular drug of abuse.**

Beta-adrenergic Blockers

Propranolol (Inderal) may have a particular usefulness in the treatment of **anxiety with marked somatic (adrenergic) symptoms** (e.g., tachycar-dia, palpitations, tremor). It is not currently FDA approved for the treat-ment of anxiety per se.

Over-the-counter Hypnotic Preparations

These agents (e.g., Sominex) contain a combination of methapyrilene (an antihistamine), scopolamine, and salicylamide. These mixtures have been shown to be **no more effective than placebos,** and run the risk of producing **anticholinergic toxicity.**

Additional Readings

AMA Drug Evaluations, 4th ed. Chicago, American Medical Association, 1980

Baldessarini RJ: Chemotherapy in Psychiatry. Cambridge, MA, Harvard University Press, 1977

Diagnostic and Statistic Manual, 3rd ed. (DSM III). Washington, DC, American Psychiatric Association, 1980

Hollister LE: Clinical Pharmacology of Psychotherapeutic Drugs. New York, Churchill Livingstone, 1978

Jefferson JW, Greist JH: Primer of Lithium Therapy. Baltimore, Williams & Wilkins, 1977

Manual of Psychiatric Therapeutics. Edited by Shader, RI. Boston, Little, Brown, 1975

Pirodsky DM: Primer of Clinical Psychopharmacology: A Practical Guide. New York, Medical Examination Publishing, 1981

Psychopharmacology, from Theory to Practice. Edited by Barchas JD, Berger PA, Ciaranello RD, Elliot GR. New York, Oxford University Press, 1977

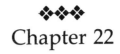

Chapter 22

Legal Issues

Franklin G. Reed

Civil Commitment

Because psychiatric patients may have distortions and disorders of consciousness and thought, their ability to make informed judgments about their own welfare can be impaired. In addition, they can become a hazard to themselves or others through violence or self-injury. Consequently, laws exist which allow the physician to initiate involuntary treatment. On one hand, civil commitment is a medical procedure for hospitalizing disturbed persons. Healing professionals are authorized to manage this process. On the other, commitment of individuals to an institution without their consent also constitutes a deprivation of their freedom. Commitment thus is also a legal procedure. Because we place a high priority on the liberty of individual citizens, the imposition of state authority even for the purpose of treatment has become a legal problem with judicial supervision of the medical process. Every state has laws enabling commitment of individual citizens dangerous to others because of mental illness.

Because the government may act as *parens patriae* (parent of the nation) it claims the right also to commit disabled persons for their own welfare even if not dangerous. Despite the theoretical and political questions raised by this relationship between the state and its citizens, the parens patriae principle justifies commitment, as it does child labor laws or regulation of hospital standards. Thus, many states commit individuals for psychiatric treatment who are mentally ill, need treatment, and (in some states) are unable to recognize that need. For example, a profoundly depressed widower, isolated and withdrawn from his family and friends, convinced that there is no reason to seek help because life will never be better, may be committed in some states.

Standards of commitability alone, however, will not ensure that justice will be done, or serious abuse avoided. Therefore, the law goes further, specifying the procedures of commitment: who may commit and under what circumstances. Some states specify that initial commitment be made by judges, while others allow commitments by physicians. Most provide a mixture of the two. In New York, for example, physicians are authorized to do the initial commitment. But they are monitored closely by the courts which have the authority to extend the commitment beyond its initial time limit of three to 60 days. **Practicing physicians must become familiar with the commitment standards and procedures of their own state.** These identify criteria for involuntary hospitalization and the specific steps which must be followed.

Limits of Treatment

Physicians do not have absolute freedom to treat patients in any manner they choose. Until the 1970s malpractice litigation was the major legal limitation on the unrestrained right of physicians to treat psychiatric patients. Since then, two new grounds for legal action have developed, namely, the right to refuse treatment and the right to treatment. Physicians once assumed that if they met the ethical and clinical standards of the profession, and avoided negligent practices, they had the right and responsibility to determine appropriate treatment for involuntary patients. In 1965, for example, damages were awarded to a patient who a New York court found should have been given medication despite his refusals, because he had been committed to the hospital. Although the defendant physician explained that he had not used drugs because the patient refused them, the court said, "We consider such a reason to be illogical, unprofessional, and not consonant with prevailing medical standards."

Right to Refuse Treatment

By 1979, with cases in Massachusetts and New Jersey (*Rogers v Okin* and *Rennie v Kline*), the courts began to find that even patients involuntarily committed for psychiatric care had the constitutional right to refuse treatment. That right, the courts held, was qualified by the risk which the treatment posed to the patient, the risks posed by not treating the patient, the availability of adequate, less restrictive treatment, and the patient's capacity to give informed consent. At this time, **this new right has not been applied in all states;** and its development and implementation are evolving. It is necessary to keep up-to-date on this issue.

Cases are establishing legal rights which did not exist before. As a result, many states are formulating administrative procedures for handling patient objections to routine psychiatric treatment. Their presence limits and constrains clinical practice in new ways.

Right to Treatment

This is another area of the law which is advancing rapidly. The most influential statement and application of this occurred in the case of *Wyatt v Stickney* in Alabama. In that case, the plaintiffs, a whole class of Alabama citizens involuntarily committed to that state's hospitals, were found to have been deprived of their liberty under the parens patriae concept. They needed treatment, but were not given it. Indeed, the basic care given to many patients in the Alabama state facilities was found by the court to be so limited that their continued retention amounted to "cruel and inhuman punishment" and a violation of due process and equal protection under the law. The Wyatt court enunciated the principle that, if a person is involuntarily committed, he must be given adequate treatment and care. After extensive hearings, that court published constitutional standards for the minimal level of care required (many of which are now incorporated in hospital accreditation criteria). These and other cases have limited the physician's right to withhold or require treatment. In addition, administrative standards are being developed for utilization review, PSRO, Medicaid/Medicare, etc.

Civil Competency

Consent for Treatment

Closely related to the right to refuse treatment is the issue of the patient's capacity to consent to it. The law assumes that individuals are competent to give or withhold such consent. Therefore, a medical or surgical patient may **not** be treated without his consent. In cases where the patient refuses to authorize necessary treatment, the physician or the hospital may go to court to determine the patient's competence. This should ordinarily be done only if it appears that the refusal is the result of a mental disorder (such as dementia), which significantly limits his ability to understand the nature of the treatment proposed, the risks of both treatment and failure to treat, or interferes with his motivation to be well (such as depression or delusions). If he is judged incompetent to consent, a third party will be appointed by the court, termed a guardian or committee, who is empowered to perform the consent function for the patient.

Competency for Other Legal Functions

Mentally ill persons may be judged incompetent to perform other legal functions as well, such as **making a will or managing their financial affairs.** Usually this problem arises in patients with severe or progressive dementia, recurrent manic–depressive disorder, and chronic schizophrenia. In dementia, the physician may often anticipate the development of symptoms such as disorientation, confusion, and memory loss, and assist the patient and family in planning to manage financial and business affairs as the disability worsens. Often, just a power of attorney can be used, in lieu of guardianship, in cases where the symptoms will prevent the patient from doing necessary business. In situations where it is necessary to limit the patient's business and financial activity (such as recurrent manic spending), or protect the patient's assets from others, the physician should recommend consultation with an attorney and a formal competency proceeding.

Competence to Stand Trial

The Sixth Amendment to the Constitution of the United States guarantees trial to a citizen accused of a crime. The defendant has a right to face his accusers and have the assistance of counsel. Because of mental illness, many persons are unable to understand the trial process or to assist their attorney. When the physician is asked to report to the court on the competency of an individual to perform a defined legal function, he must understand the legal standard in his jurisdiction for that act. The question before the court is precise: at this time, is the defendant able to stand trial? After examining the patient, the physician should be able to describe how the defendant's symptoms interefere with his ability to act effectively in the trial process. Based on that description, the court will make its (own) decision.

Insanity as a Defense

Examining for competency to stand trial is different from examining for insanity as a defense. To determine insanity one must assess the mental status of the defendant at some time in the past and judge whether or not it affected his ability to perform knowingly, rationally, and wrongfully the **specific** alleged criminal acts. **Insane is a legal term,** not a psychiatric one. As with civil commitment, **each state** defines the kind and degree of mental impairment which must be present before a mentally ill person may be excused as "insane" for committing otherwise criminal acts. When examining a defendant for sanity, the defendant's mental illness as well as the specific acts of which he is accused must be understood. Report of symptoms must be relevant to that state's definition of sanity–insanity. A person may have been insane, yet be competent to stand trial. Conversely, a patient may now be incompetent to stand trial but have been sane when committing the criminal act. **It is the law, not medicine, which defines both competency and sanity.** The purpose of the psychiatric examination is to determine if the defendant had or has a mental illness and if so, if the level of the symptoms reaches the legal standard of that state.

Conclusions

Whether deciding on commitment, judging a patient's right to receive or refuse treatment, or determining competence or sanity, the physician may rely on a precise interpretation of the law to guide his conduct and decision. **There are many more people who are mentally ill than persons who are committable, incompetent, or insane.** The law protects them. In general, the law is relatively reasonable and remarkably flexible in its application, despite recent trends towards increasing rigidity and intrusiveness. Attention to the guidance of peers and awareness of new information are vital; but the careful listening to the needs and wishes of patients is the most effective and reliable guide to practice.

Additional Readings

Brooks AD: Law, Psychiatry and The Mental Health System. Boston, Little, Brown, 1974

Roth LH, Meisel A, Lidz CW: Tests of competency to consent to treatment. Am J Psychiatry 134:279–284, 1977

Roth LH: A commitment law for patients, doctors, and lawyers. Am J Psychiatry 136:1121–1127, 1979

Stone A: Recent mental health litigation: A critical perspective. Am J Psychiatry 134:273–279, 1977

The right to refuse treatment (special section). Am J Psychiatry 137:329–358, 1980

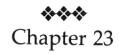

Chapter 23

The Referral Process

Magnus Lakovics

Many patients with psychiatric disturbances can be managed and treated by nonpsychiatrists. Frequently, chronic schizophrenic patients on maintenance medication, manic–depressive patients, mildly or chronically depressed patients on antidepressants, acute adjustment disorders, medical problems in which psychological factors are prominent, and a number of other psychiatric problems can be safely and effectively cared for in the ambulatory medical setting.

However it is important that the physician maintain a close relationship with a psychiatrist colleague to whom he can turn for informal advice, as well as formal consultation or referral for treatment. It is often assumed that the only effective consultation is through referral. This is not the case. A few brief words of advice about a case may be all that is necessary. Referral often occurs after a physician has extended his best efforts which have met with failure over a prolonged period without consultation. These patients may feel they are abandoned, criticized, being called liars about their symptoms, and betrayed. A typical case is the hypochondriacal or somatizing patient who is "polypharmacized" to the extreme. When none of this is effective, then he is told to "go see a psychiatrist."

Each chapter in this book has clarified the circumstances under which psychiatric referral should be made. However, several other aspects of referral need to be considered. **How should patients be referred for further specialized psychiatric treatment? Where should they be referred? What can they expect?**

Psychiatric referral can be a traumatic affair angrily rejected or only grudgingly pursued; or it can be helpful, gratefully received, and uneventful if properly undertaken.

If the physician wishes his patient to get effective psychiatric care he must be able to make the referral in a way that diminishes the patient's fear and stimulates motivation for compliance. Two factors are important in this respect. One is the **physician's attitude.** The other is **the manner in which a patient is referred.**

Attitude can be the greatest facilitator or impediment to psychiatric referral. Attitude is important because patients often respond to this rather than any overt statements being made. If the physician does not believe a patient with psychiatric disturbance is suffering or that his symptoms are not important or even "real," but that he is malingering, lying, or is "just a complainer," the patient will feel as if he is being referred to a psychiatrist because his doctor dislikes and no longer wants to be troubled with him. He will feel rejected and may well not seek out further help until he gets worse. Similarly, if the physician feels that psychiatric problems are incurable, or psychiatric treatment is worthless, his patient is likely to pick up this same view and is unlikely to pursue the referral. In contrast, a positive, realistic attitude conveyed along with interest and involvement in the referral process will enhance motivation and compliance.

If a good doctor–patient relationship has been established, an in-depth, empathic, and comprehensive interview and psychiatric examination have outlined the problems accurately, the manner of referral is second nature. The process continues from the evaluation as a simple, honest, and open discussion of referral, rather than an announcement. More often than not, the patient himself will see the necessity for this and desire it. He may even have thought of this earlier but may have been unwilling to make the first move because of embarrassment, shame, or fear. Often doctors are concerned that a patient will be insulted by psychiatric referral. This is a myth. If it is done with empathy and sensitivity, usually he will appreciate the genuine concern to find some solution to what may seem an unsolvable problem. Of course, an occasional patient reacts negatively either with fear or anger. The first step is to note and explore these feelings. Once they become understood, almost invariably they can be dealt with by direct reassurance and explanation. They usually arise from prejudice, ignorance, or simple uncertainty. The physician can ordinarily educate such a patient with little difficulty, if he is supportive and takes the time.

Once a clinical decision has been made (see Chapter 13) concerning the referral of a patient for outpatient or inpatient psychiatric care, what can the referring physician expect from the psychiatrist, mental health professional, and outpatient or inpatient service?

Common Sources for Outpatient Psychiatric Referral

Private Psychiatrists

Psychiatrists may have many differing orientations to practice. Some have only office practices. If a patient has been hospitalized in the past, or it looks as if hospitalization may be necessary in the future, referral to this type of psychiatrist may not serve future needs well. Other psychiatrists are based on inpatient services and devote a major portion of their time to hospital work. They frequently provide ongoing care and treatment for seriously disturbed individuals on an inpatient and outpatient basis. They may not be as willing to provide long-term outpatient treatment to less-disturbed individuals. Still others have office practices but work with the proviso that if their patients require hospitalization, they will continue treating them there. Thus when referring it is helpful to know and communicate the patient's current needs, and what may be anticipated in the near future. A patient may be lost in the shuffle if the practice style of the psychiatrist and the patient's needs are mismatched.

Other Mental Health Professionals

A number of psychologists, social workers, counselors, etc. conduct private practices. Each of these professionals have different skills with varying styles of practice. Clinical psychologists are expert in psychometric testing, and some in psychotherapy as well. Others may be experts in behavior therapy. Social workers may (or may not) be trained in psychotherapy; and a number of these have special skills in treating a family group. Others have more limited skills, providing supportive counseling and practical help with socioeconomic problems. Sexual counselors may provide skilled help in their field. But the physician must first be sure (by his own examination or psychiatric consultation) that the problem is not reflective of deeper conflicts or psychopathology requiring a psychiatrist. Ordinarily, any patient who has significant medical problems, requires medication for his psychiatric disorder, or presents problems of differential diagnosis should be referred only to a psychiatrist. This may be for consultation, with only one question being posed about the preferred treatment modality or further referral. It is important to find out what specific skills a given professional has before referral.

Community Mental Health Center

Community mental health centers (CMHCs) are principally staffed by psychologists, social workers, and other mental health professionals. Psychiatrists work as consultants, and treat inpatients, if the CMHC has an inpatient unit. These centers are frequently busy so that nonemergent cases may have a long wait. **Do not assume that a physician will see a patient referred to a CMHC.** CMHCs often offer a wide range of services such as day care or partial hospitalization; occasionally drug abuse and alcoholism programs; outpatient psychotherapeutic treatment; vocational rehabilitation, rarely sheltered workshops; access to halfway houses (staffed but not treatment-oriented facilities); and a variety of activity programs. Patients may be required to be residents of a particular geographic area to be eligible for care.

State Hospitals

State hospitals may have outreach clinics, which often are similar to CMHCs. Some may be affiliated with a neighboring CMHC.

Other Public Services

These include pastoral counseling centers, health maintenance organizations, nonprofit subsidized clinics, university center clinics, college health services, Veterans Administration (VA) mental hygiene clinics, etc. Often they have specific criteria for admission: income, organizational membership, diagnosis, etc. It is important to know these criteria since an inappropriate referral may lead to a patient getting lost in the "referral maze." It is also important to know what groups of professionals serve on their staff, for the reasons already noted.

Common Sources for Inpatient Psychiatric Referral

Referral for inpatient psychiatric services is usually best handled by **direct contact with the psychiatrist to whom the patient is being referred or the admitting psychiatrist of the service.** If this is not possible, a responsible psychiatrist affiliated with the particular institution should be contacted. Simply telling a disturbed patient to "sign himself in" to a psychiatric institution is poor practice.

Psychiatric inpatient units vary in services they offer. Again, familiarity with what these services are is an important factor in deciding on the referral. Three basic types of inpatient units form the crux of inpatient psychiatric care in this country.

General Hospital Psychiatric Units

Units located in general hospitals (private, VA, county, etc.) generally provide acute treatment services with a short length of stay (usually up to 30 days, but sometimes longer). **Patients are usually admitted and**

cared for by a psychiatrist who may be in private practice or be hospital employed (who may care for some or all of the patients but also have administrative duties). In some cases, unit policies may require that permission be obtained from the psychiatrist director of the unit before a patient is accepted (an administrative arrangement similar to some medical and surgical ICUs). General hospital psychiatric units offer 24-hour nursing care, provide milieu treatment, group therapy, and of course treatment from the patient's own psychiatrist. On a few units, psychologists may admit patients under the supervision of the psychiatrist. In some cases, a psychiatric social worker may be employed to work with the patients. Often, additional services such as activity therapy, art therapy, occupational therapy, and vocational rehabilitation are provided. **Units vary in whether they will admit only voluntary patients or involuntary (committed) patients** as well. Three advantages of hospitalization on a general hospital psychiatric unit are proximity to home and family, lower stigma, and the immediate availability of consultants and laboratory facilities.

Freestanding Psychiatric Hospital Facilities

This category includes both private, public (county, state, federal) hospitals and those community mental health centers which have inpatient units. Most of these provide both acute and chronic care. Lengths of stay vary from short (days to weeks) to intermediate (weeks to months) to long stay (months to years). Many freestanding facilities include specialized units for programs such as behavior therapy, alcohol detoxification and treatment, drug and adolescent treatment, rehabilitation, and skilled nursing care. In some of these facilities, admissions are only by referral through an outpatient facility. Others admit patients only after screening by a psychiatrist, psychologist, or social worker on their staff. Some require that a patient meet certain criteria, such as being a state resident, veteran, or living within a fixed geographic catchment area. With the exception of CMHCs and private hospitals, most of these facilities are located away from major cities. This separates the patient from his family, friends, and community. Most, but not all, will take involuntary patients. Because these are specialized hospitals, additional services such as activity therapy, art therapy, occupational therapy, and vocational rehabilitation specific for psychiatric patients are usually available, and may be integrated specifically into the treatment programs. This is one of their major advantages. Another is the usual close working relationship with outpatient facilities. This may be particularly important to follow-up care of chronic patients. Some disadvantages include their location, and reduced availability of quality general medical care (consultants, laboratory services, etc.). Of course, some have arrangements with local general hospitals; or have a "med-surg" unit on the grounds. In addition, some of the larger, poorly funded public facilities have inadequate numbers and quality of staff.

Conclusions

The physician who conducts the process of referral as a therapeutic act, in a positive and skilled manner, will find that his patients are most likely to respond to his advice and to benefit most from the ensuing treatment. In addition, he must be familiar with the particular skills and services available from the psychiatrist (or other professional) or facility he chooses. If he is reasonably fortunate in his locale, a variety of services are available. But **the key is to develop a close professional relationship with one or more psychiatrist colleagues,** preferably someone to whom he can turn for informal advice as well as consultation and referral. If one person is chosen, it should be a competent general psychiatrist who either conducts or is directly familiar with different types of treatment for various patient groups, and with other professional services available in the community.

Additional Readings

Lazare A, Eisenthal S, Wasserman NL: The customer approach to patienthood. Arch Gen Psychiatry 32:553–558, 1975

Rogawski AS, Edmundson B: Factors affecting the outcome of psychiatric inter-agency referral. Am J Psychiatry 127:925–934, 1971

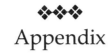

Appendix

The DSM III Classification:
Axes I and II

Axis I

*Disorders Usually
First Evident in Infancy,
Childhood, or Adolescence*

Mental retardation:

317.0(x)* Mild mental
          retardation
318.0(x)   Moderate mental
          retardation
318.1(x)   Severe mental
          retardation
318.2(x)   Profound mental
          retardation
319.0(x)   Unspecified
          mental retardation

Code in fifth digit: 1 = with other behavioral symptoms (requiring attention or treatment and that are not part of another disorder, 0 =

without other behavioral symptoms.

Attention deficit disorder:

314.01 with hyperactivity
314.00 without hyperactivity
314.80 residual type

Conduct disorder:

312.00 undersocialized,
        aggressive
312.10 undersocialized,
        nonaggressive
312.23 socialized, aggressive
312.2.1 socialized,
        nonaggressive
312.90 atypical

Anxiety disorders of childhood or adolescence:

309.21 Separation anxiety
        disorder

*An x indicates the use of various fifth digit codes, which provide additional detail about the nature of the disorder.

313.21   Avoidant disorder of
         childhood or
         adolescence
313.00   Overanxious disorder

Other disorders of infancy, childhood, or adolescence:
313.89   Reactive attachment
         disorder of infancy
313.22   Schizoid disorder of
         childhood or
         adolescence
313.23   Elective mutism
313.81   Oppositional disorder
313.82   Identity disorder

Eating disorders:
307.10   Anorexia nervosa
307.51   Bulimia
307.52   Pica
307.53   Rumination disorder of
         infancy
307.50   Atypical eating disorder

Stereotyped movement disorders:
307.21   Transient tic disorder
307.22   Chronic motor tic
         disorder
307.23   Tourette's disorder
307.20   Atypical tic disorder
307.30   Atypical stereotyped
         movement disorder

Other disorders with physical
manifestations:
307.00   Stuttering
307.60   Functional enuresis
307.70   Functional encopresis
307.46   Sleepwalking disorder
307.46   Sleep terror disorder

Pervasive developmental disorders:
299.0(x)   Infantile autism
299.9(x)   Childhood onset
           pervasive
           developmental
           disorder
299.8(x)   Atypical

Code in fifth digit: 0 = full syndrome present, 1 = residual state.

Organic Mental Disorders

Section 1. Organic mental disorders whose etiology or pathophysiological process is listed below.

Dementias arising in the senium
   and presenium.
Primary degenerative dementia,
   senile onset
290.30   with delirium
290.20   with delusions
290.21   with depression
290.00   uncomplicated

Code in fifth digit: 1 = with delirium, 2 = with delusions, 3 = with
depression, 0 = uncomplicated.

290.1(x)   Primary degenerative
           dementia presenile
           onset
290.4(x)   Multi-infarct dementia

Substance-induced
           Alcohol
303.00   intoxication
291.40   idiosyncratic intoxication
291.80   withdrawal
291.00   withdrawal delirium
291.30   hallucinosis
291.10   amnestic disorder

Code severity of dementia in fifth digit: 1 = mild, 2 = moderate, 3 = severe, 0 = unspecified.

291.2(x)   Dementia associated with alcoholism

Code in fifth digit as for other dementias.

Barbiturate or similarly acting sedative or hypnotic

305.40   intoxication
292.00   withdrawal
292.00   withdrawal delirium
292.83   amnestic disorder

Opioid

305.50   intoxication
292.00   withdrawal

Cocaine

305.60   intoxication

Amphetamine or similarly acting sympathomimetic

305.70   intoxication
292.81   delirium
292.11   delusional disorder
292.00   withdrawal

Phencyclidine (PCP) or similarly acting arylcyclohexylamine

305.90   intoxication
292.81   delirium
292.90   mixed organic mental disorder

Hallucinogen

305.30   hallucinosis
292.11   delusional disorder
292.84   affective disorder

Cannabis

305.20   intoxication
292.11   delusional disorder

Tobacco

292.00   withdrawal

Caffeine

305.90   intoxication

Other or unspecified substance

305.90   intoxication
292.00   withdrawal
292.81   delirium
292.82   dementia
292.83   amnestic disorder
292.11   delusional disorder
292.12   hallucinosis
292.84   affective disorder
292.89   personality disorder
292.90   atypical or mixed organic mental disorder

Section 2. Organic brain syndromes whose etiology or pathophysiological process is either noted as an additional diagnosis outside the mental disorders or is unknown.

293.00   Delirium
294.10   Dementia
294.00   Amnestic syndrome
293.81   Organic delusional syndrome
293.82   Organic hallucinosis
293.83   Organic affective syndrome
310.10   Organic personality syndrome
294.80   Atypical or mixed organic brain syndrome

Substance Use Disorders

305.0(x) Alcohol abuse

303.9(x) Alcohol dependence (Alcoholism)

305.4(x) Barbiturate or similarly acting sedative or hypnotic abuse

304.1(x) Barbiturate or similarly acting sedative or hypnotic dependence

305.5(x) Opioid abuse

304.0(x) Opioid dependence

305.6(x) Cocaine abuse

305.7(x) Amphetamine or similarly acting sympathomimetic abuse

304.4(x) Amphetamine or similarly acting sympathomimetic dependence

305.9(x) Phencyclidine (PCP) or similarly acting arylcyclohexylamine abuse

305.3(x) Hallucinogen abuse

305.2(x) Cannabis abuse

304.3(x) Cannabis dependence

305.1(x) Tobacco dependence

305.9(x) Other, mixed, or unspecified substance abuse

304.6(x) Other specified substance dependence

304.9(x) Unspecified substance dependence

304.7(x) Dependence on combination of opioid and other nonalcoholic substance

304.8(x) Dependence on combination of substances, excluding opioids and alcohol

Code in fifth digit: 1 = continuous, 2 = episodic, 3 = in remission, 0 = unspecified.

Schizophrenic Disorders

Schizophrenia

295.1(x) disorganized

295.2(x) catatonic

295.3(x) paranoid

295.9(x) undifferentiated

295.6(x) residual

Code in fifth digit: 1 = subchronic, 2 = chronic, 3 = subchronic with acute exacerbation, 4 = chronic with acute exacerbation, 5 = in remission, 0 = unspecified.

Paranoid Disorders

297.10 Paranoia

297.30 Shared paranoid disorder

298.30 Acute paranoid disorder

297.90 Atypical paranoid disorder

Psychotic Disorders Not Elsewhere Classified

295.40 Schizophreniform disorder

298.80 Brief reactive psychosis

295.70 Schizoaffective disorder

298.90 Atypical psychosis

Affective Disorders

Major affective disorders:

   Bipolar disorder
296.6(x) mixed
296.4(x) manic
296.5(x) depressed

   Major depression
296.2(x) single episode
296.3(x) recurrent

Code major depressive episode in fifth digit: 6 = in remission, 4 = with psychotic features (the unofficial fifth digit 7 may be used instead to indicate that the psychotic features are mood incongruent), 3 = with melancholia, 2 = without melancholia, 0 = unspecified.

Code manic or mixed episode in fifth digit: 6 = in remission, 4 = with psychotic features (the unofficial fifth digit 7 may be used instead to indicate that the psychotic features are mood incongruent), 2 = without psychotic features, 0 = unspecified.

Other specific affective disorders:
301.13 Cyclothymic disorder
300.40 Dysthymic disorder
           (or Depressive neurosis)

Atypical affective disorders:
296.70 Atypical bipolar disorder
296.82 Atypical depression

Anxiety Disorders

Phobic disorders (or Phobic neuroses:
300.21 Agoraphobia with panic
           attacks
300.22 Agoraphobia without
           panic attacks

300.23 Social phobia
300.29 Simple phobia

Anxiety states (or Anxiety neuroses):
300.01 Panic disorder
300.02 Generalized anxiety
           disorder
300.30 Obsessive–compulsive
           disorder (or Obsessive–
           compulsive neurosis)

Posttraumatic stress disorder:
308.30 acute
309.81 chronic or delayed
300.00 Atypical anxiety disorder

Somatoform Disorders
300.81 Somatization disorder
300.11 Conversion disorder (or
           Hysterical neurosis,
           conversion type)
307.80 Psychogenic pain
           disorder
300.70 Hypochondriasis (or
           Hypochondriacal
           neurosis)
300.70 Atypical somatoform
           disorder

Dissociative Disorders
(Or Hysterical Neuroses,
Dissociative Type)
300.12 Psychogenic amnesia
300.13 Psychogenic fugue
300.14 Multiple personality
300.60 Depersonalization
           disorder (or
           Depersonalization
           neurosis)
300.15 Atypical dissociative
           disorder

Psychosexual Disorders

Gender identity disorders:

302.5(x)   Transsexualism

302.60   Gender identity disorder
of childhood

302.85   Atypical gender identity
disorder

Indicate sexual history in the fifth
digit of Transsexualism code: 1 =
asexual, 2 = homosexual, 3 = het-
erosexual, 0 = unspecified.

Paraphilias:

302.81   Fetishism

302.30   Transvestism

302.10   Zoophilia

302.20   Pedophilia

302.40   Exhibitionism

302.82   Voyeurism

302.83   Sexual masochism

302.84   Sexual sadism

302.90   Atypical paraphilia

Psychosexual dysfunctions:

302.71   Inhibited sexual desire

302.72   Inhibited sexual
excitement

302.73   Inhibited female orgasm

302.74   Inhibited male orgasm

302.75   Premature ejaculation

302.76   Functional dyspareunia

306.51   Functional vaginismus

302.70   Atypical psychosexual
dysfunction

Other psychosexual disorders:

302.00   Ego-dystonic
homosexuality

302.89   Psychosexual disorder
not elsewhere
classified

Factitious Disorders

300.16   Factitious disorder with
psychological
symptoms

301.51   Chronic factitious
disorder with physical
symptoms

300.19   Atypical factitious
disorder with physical
symptoms

*Disorders of Impulse Control Not
Elsewhere Classified*

312.31   Pathological gambling

312.32   Kleptomania

312.33   Pyromania

312.34   Intermittent explosive
disorder

312.35   Isolated explosive
disorder

312.39   Atypical impulse control
disorder

Adjustment Disorder

309.00   with depressed mood

309.24   with anxious mood

309.28   with mixed emotional
features

309.30   with disturbance of
conduct

309.40   with mixed disturbance
of emotions and
conduct

309.23   with work (or academic)
inhibition

309.83   with withdrawal

309.90   with atypical features

Psychological Factors Affecting Physical Condition

Specify physical condition on Axis III.

316.00   Psychological factors affecting physical condition

V Codes for Conditions Not Attributable to a Mental Disorder That Are a Focus of Attention or Treatment

V65.20   Malingering

V62.89   Borderline intellectual functioning

V71.01   Adult antisocial behavior

V71.02   Childhood or adolescent antisocial behavior

V62.30   Academic problem

V62.20   Occupational problem

V62.82   Uncomplicated bereavement

V15.81   Noncompliance with medical treatment

V62.89   Phase of life problem or other life circumstance problem

V61.10   Marital problem

V61.20   Parent–child problem

V61.80   Other specified family circumstances

V62.81   Other interpersonal problem

Axis II

Specific Developmental Disorders

315.00   Developmental reading disorder

315.10   Developmental arithmetic disorder

315.31   Developmental language disorder

315.39   Developmental articulation disorder

315.50   Mixed specific developmental disorder

315.90   Atypical specific developmental disorder

Personality Disorders

301.00   Paranoid

301.20   Schizoid

301.22   Schizotypal

301.50   Histrionic

301.81   Narcissistic

301.70   Antisocial

301.83   Borderline

301.82   Avoidant

301.60   Dependent

301.40   Compulsive

301.84   Passive–Aggressive

301.89   Atypical, mixed, or other personality disorder

Index